KT-514-332

BMA

British Medical Association

Home
DOCTOR

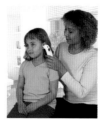

Wyggeston QE I

00597505

LONDON, NEW YORK, MUNICH, MELBOURNE, DELHI

BRITISH MEDICAL ASSOCIATION
Chairman of the Council Dr Hamish Meldrum
Treasurer Dr David Pickersgill
Chairman of the Representative Body Dr Peter Bennie

DORLING KINDERSLEY
Project Editor Esther Ripley
Editors Katie John, Alyson Lacewing
Managing Editors Julie Oughton, Martyn Page
Project Art Editors Sue Caws, Isabel de Cordova
Managing Art Editors Louise Dick, Marianne Markham
Picture Researchers Romaine Werblow, Claire Bowers, Juliet Duff, Carolyn Clerkin
Production Editor Phil Sergeant
Production Controller Hema Gohil
Associate Publisher Liz Wheeler
Publisher Jonathan Metcalf
Art Director Bryn Walls
Additional Design Inperspective Ltd., Ist Floor, Exmouth House, 3–11 Pine Street, London EC1R 0JH

Second edition edited for Dorling Kindersley by Martyn Page
Child Health Reviewer Ann Peters RGN, Health Visitor

Published in the UK by Dorling Kindersley Limited, 80 Strand, London WC2R ORL
A Penguin Company
Second edition 2009

4 6 8 10 9 7 5 3

The *British Medical Association Home Doctor* provides information on a wide range of medical topics, and every effort has been made to ensure that the information in this book is accurate. The information in this book will be relevant to the majority of people but may not be applicable in each individual case so you are therefore advised to obtain expert medical advice for specific information on personal health matters. Never disregard expert medical advice or delay in receiving treatment due to information obtained from this book. The naming of any product, treatment, or organization in this book does not imply endorsement by the BMA, author, or publisher, nor does the omission of any such names indicate disapproval. The BMA, author, and publisher do not accept any legal responsibility for any personal injury or other damage or loss arising from any use or misuse of the information and advice in this book.

Copyright © 2004, 2009 Dorling Kindersley Ltd, London
Text copyright © 2004, 2009 Michael Peters
The author has asserted his moral right to be identified as the author of this work.

All rights reserved. No part of this publication may be reproduced, stored in a retrieval system, or transmitted in any form or by any means, electronic, mechanical, photocopying, recording, or otherwise, without the prior written permission of the copyright owner.

A CIP catalogue record for this book is available from the British Library
ISBN 978 1 4053 4201 8
Colour reproduction by Colourscan, Singapore
Printed and bound in China by Hung Hing Offset Printing Company Ltd

Discover more at
www.dk.com

BMA

British Medical Association

Home
DOCTOR

Dr Michael Peters

A Dorling Kindersley Book

Foreword

Acc. No.

00597505

Class No.
616.024 PET

People today are more aware of health issues than ever before, but they are frequently confronted with a bewildering array of self-help advice. There is often little guidance through this maze, leaving many people confused about when and who to ask for help, and sometimes suffering because they do not want to bother their doctor with "trivial" complaints.

As a GP for many years, I have always thought it is important to empower people by giving them clear information to enable them to make sensible decisions about their health. I also feel that people should be better informed so that they can make lifestyle changes that can help prevent disease. In writing *Home Doctor* I have tried to put this into practice, covering over 150 common conditions for which home treatment is often appropriate. In each article, I have given guidance on identifying your condition and deciding whether self-help is suitable, and advice on practical help and treatment. This guidance and advice should give you the confidence to treat minor conditions yourself or, in the event of serious illness or injury, to know when you should see your own doctor.

I have endeavoured to make this book simple to use. At the top of each page, the topic is briefly but clearly explained, and advice is given in easy-to-follow steps. The warning signs of serious illness are clearly marked. You are also told at the outset when you can treat a condition yourself or if you need to see a doctor. Treatment options involve practical techniques and tips, conventional treatments, and a few tried-and-tested complementary therapies, making this book more holistic than many in its approach.

A range of drug and natural remedies is suggested in this book, with more information – such as brand names, how to use them, possible side effects, and precautions – given in a special section at the end of the book. There are a vast number of treatments available in pharmacies and health stores, but I have confined myself to those that I feel are most likely to be effective. Naturally, however, there will be omissions or alternatives that may be just as suitable. Information about drugs is particularly important as there are an increasing number of more powerful drugs that were previously only available with a prescription from a doctor, but are now available over the counter. These drugs are generally sold in lower dosages and/or shorter courses, and sometimes only for certain age groups, than those on prescription. As far as possible, I have used a similar evidence-based approach in choosing natural remedies, with the occasional addition of a soothing herbal tea or oil that may help and is unlikely to cause harm.

This second edition of the book has been thoroughly revised and updated. As well as deletion of treatments not now thought to be helpful and/or to have unacceptable side effects, there are new additions, including antibiotic eye drops to treat bacterial conjunctivitis and wart freezing preparations to treat warts and verrucas. The First Aid section at the back of the book has been updated to include current guidelines. This section could prove invaluable in an emergency, when medical help may be some time or distance away.

In researching and writing this book, I have tried to create a simple home reference that can be turned to when any family member is unwell or needs medical advice. However, a book can only give general guidance and is no substitute for professional advice. When you can't find an answer here, or are in doubt about a medical condition, you should see your own doctor.

Dr Michael Peters

Contents

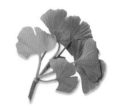

How to use this book 8

Symptom finder 9

COMMON CONDITIONS 11–152

General symptoms

Fever 12

Excessive sweating 13

Itching 14

Tiredness 15

Hangover 16

Difficulty sleeping 17

Jet lag 18

Feeling faint or dizzy 19

Stress 20

Feeling depressed 22

Panic attacks 24

Poor memory 25

Infectious diseases

Mumps 26

Rubella 27

Glandular fever 28

Measles 29

Influenza 30

Whooping cough 31

Chickenpox 32

Shingles 33

Skin, hair, and nail problems

Impetigo 34

Scabies 35

Hives 36

Acne 37

Eczema 38

Psoriasis 39

Rosacea 40

Dry skin 41

Corns and calluses 42

Warts and verrucas 43

Athlete's foot and jock itch 44

Boils 45

Heat rash and sunburn 46

Ringworm 48

Dandruff 49

Lice 50

Unwanted or ingrowing hair 51

Hair thinning and hair loss 52

Disfigured or brittle nails 53

Nailbiting 54

Ingrowing toenail 55

Eye and ear problems

Itchy eyes 56

Dry eyes 57

Conjunctivitis 58

Stye 59

Contact lens problems 60

Foreign object in the eye 61

Black eye 62

Earwax 63

Earache 64

Swimmer's ear 65

Popping ears 66

Tinnitus 67

Foreign object in the ear 68

Mouth, nose, and throat problems

Chapped or cracked lips 69

Cold sore 70

Mouth ulcer 71

Bad breath 72

Sore mouth or tongue 73

Bleeding gums 74

Toothache and sensitive teeth 75

Knocked-out tooth 76

Blocked or runny nose 77

Common cold 78

Sinusitis 79

Hay fever 80

Sore throat 81

Hoarseness and loss of voice 82

Nosebleed 83

Snoring 84

Head, back, and limb problems

Headache 85

Migraine 86

Stiff or sore neck 87

Lower back pain 88

Shoulder pain 90

Tennis or golfer's elbow 91

Hip pain 92

Knee pain 93

Leg cramps 94

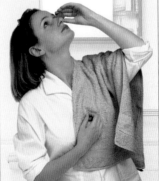

Wyggeston QE1 College
Library

Varicose veins	95
Swollen ankles	96
Foot pain	97
Bunions	98
Painful heel	99
Cold fingers and toes	100

Chest and abdominal problems

Hiccups	101
Coughing	102
Wheezing	103
Acute bronchitis	104
Palpitations	105
Indigestion	106
Heartburn	107
Bloating and flatulence	108
Nausea and vomiting	109
Motion sickness	110
Irritable bowel syndrome	111
Hernia	112
Food intolerance	113
Food poisoning	114
Constipation	115
Diarrhoea	116
Piles	117
Itchy anus	118

Men's problems

Painful scrotum	119
Painful penis	120
Urinary problems	121
Erectile dysfunction (impotence)	122
Premature ejaculation	123

Women's problems

Breast pain and lumpy breasts	124
Cracked nipples	126
Premenstrual syndrome	127

Painful periods	128
Menopausal problems	129
Cystitis	130
Poor bladder control	131
Vaginal discharge	132
Genital irritation	133
Painful intercourse	134

Children's problems

Fever	135
Diarrhoea and vomiting	136
Threadworms	137
Croup	138

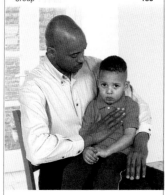

Bedwetting	139
Earache	140
Temper tantrums	141

Problems in babies

Fever	142
Diarrhoea and vomiting	143
Feeding problems	144
Sleep problems	146
Colic	148
Excessive crying	149
Spots and rashes	150
Cradle cap	151
Nappy rash	152

FIRST AID · 153–174

First aid essentials/first aid kit	154
Blisters	155
Cuts, grazes, and splinters	156
Severe bleeding	157
Insect bites and stings	158
Anaphylactic shock	159
Sprains and strains	160
Fractures and dislocations	161
Head injuries	162
Eye injuries	163
Burns and scalds	164
Shock	165
Seizures	166
Febrile seizures	167
Unconsciousness	168
Recovery position	169
CPR (adults)	170
CPR (babies and children)	171
Choking	172
Swallowed poisons	174

A–Z OF DRUG AND NATURAL REMEDIES · 175–189

Index	190
Acknowledgments	192

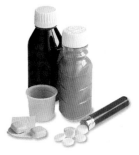

How to use this book

Home Doctor is divided into three main sections. The first, Common Conditions, is the core of the book, providing detailed advice on home treatment for a wide range of everyday disorders and complaints. The second section, First Aid, describes basic first-aid treatment for minor and more serious emergencies; and the final A–Z of Drug and Natural Remedies supplies further information on remedies suggested in articles.

Common Conditions

is divided into general symptoms; infectious diseases; groups of disorders such as eye and ear problems; and problems specific to men, women, children, and babies.

Summary of the symptoms of an illness and who it affects helps you identify the problem

What you can do yourself advises on treatment. Icons direct you to Drug remedies, Natural remedies, and Practical technique and tips boxes.

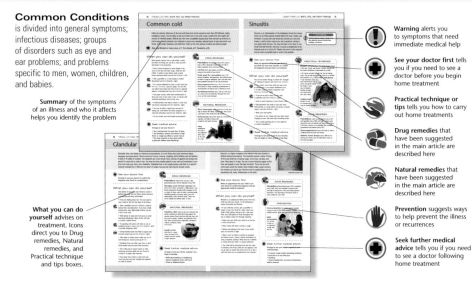

Warning alerts you to symptoms that need immediate medical help

See your doctor first tells you if you need to see a doctor before you begin home treatment

Practical technique or tips tells you how to carry out home treatments

Drug remedies that have been suggested in the main article are described here

Natural remedies that have been suggested in the main article are described here

Prevention suggests ways to help prevent the illness or recurrences

Seek further medical advice tells you if you need to see a doctor following home treatment

First Aid provides basic first-aid advice for minor mishaps and injuries, and step-by-step techniques to help you deal with serious injuries and emergencies.

Warning alerts you to when you need to call an ambulance

Summary of the injury or emergency helps you decide how to act

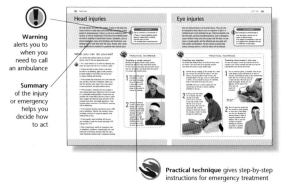

Practical technique gives step-by-step instructions for emergency treatment

A-Z of Drug and Natural Remedies

gives information, such as brand names, side effects, and precautions, for the treatments suggested in articles and general advice on using them safely.

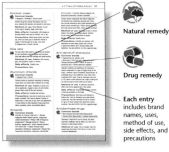

Natural remedy

Drug remedy

Each entry includes brand names, uses, method of use, side effects, and precautions

Symptom finder

Knowing exactly what is wrong when you are feeling unwell is not always easy. Individual symptoms can be caused by a variety of different illnesses, and some disorders produce surprising effects on the body that seem unrelated to the initial problem. If you are unsure which article to consult, use this symptom finder as a starting point. Each symptom listed has page references that take you to the articles in which it occurs.

A
Abdomen
    bloated 106, 107, 108, 111, 113,
        115, 116, 127
    cramps in 111, 114, 115, 116, 128, 136
    noises in 108
    pain or discomfort in 106, 108, 111, 112,
        113, 119, 130, 148, 174
Allergic reactions 38, 80, 103, 113, 150, 159
Anus
    bleeding from 117
    itchy 117, 118, 137
Anxiety 20–1, 24, 127, 159
Appetite
    increased 22–3
    loss of 18, 20–1, 22–3, 28, 116, 135, 142
Arms, pain in 87, 90, 91

B
Back
    arched or rigid 166, 167
    pain 87, 88–9, 111, 128
Bad breath 72
Bad taste in mouth 79, 107
Bald patches 52
Bedwetting 139
Belching 106, 108, 111
Bites and stings, from insects 158, 159
Bleeding
    from anus 117
    from nose 83
    severe 157, 161, 162
Blisters 32, 33, 46–7, 70, 120, 155, 164
Blurred vision 61
Bone injury 161
Bottom, sore 88–9, 92, 117, 118, 137
Bowels, feeling of fullness in 111, 117
Breastfeeding difficulty 126, 144–5
Breasts
    lumpy 124–5, 127
    painful 124–5, 127
Breath
    holding 141
    shortness of 24
Breathing
    difficulty 31, 103, 159, 172
    noisy 31, 84, 101, 138
    rapid and/or shallow 24, 110, 165
    stopped 84, 141, 167, 170–1
Bruising
    around eye 62, 163
    on limb 160, 161
Burns 164, 174

C
Chest
    pain 24
    tight feeling in 103
Chills 12
Colic 148
Confusion/disorientation 18, 25, 162, 166
Consciousness, loss of 159, 162, 164, 165,
    166, 167, 168–9, 170–1, 173, 174
Constipation 111, 115, 127
Cough
    dry 29, 30, 78, 80, 81, 102, 107, 138
    with mucus (phlegm) 102, 104
Cracked lips 69
Cramps
    leg 94
    menstrual 128
Crying, excessive 141, 148, 149
Cuts and grazes 156, 162

D
Dehydration 13, 114, 116, 136, 142, 143
Dementia 25
Depression 20–1, 22–3, 127, 129, 135
Diarrhoea (loose stools) 18, 111, 113, 114,
    116, 128, 136, 143
Dizziness 16, 19, 24, 63, 110, 114

E
Ears
    aching or pain in 63, 64, 65, 66, 140
    discharge from 64, 65, 140
    earwax, excess 63
    full or blocked feeling in 63, 65, 66
    itchy or irritated 63, 65, 68
    noises in 63, 66, 67
Ejaculation, premature 123
Erection difficulty 122
Exhaustion 30
Eyelids, sore 40, 59
Eyes
    bloodshot 163
    blurred vision 61
    debris in 61, 163
    discharge from 56, 58
    dry 57
    itchy 56, 58, 80
    pain around 62, 79, 85, 86
    red 29, 56, 58, 60, 61, 80
    sensitive to light 57, 86
    sore or irritated 30, 40, 56, 57, 60, 61, 62, 163
    swollen 62, 163
    watering 58, 60, 61, 80, 163

F
Face
    pain 79
    swollen 26, 159
Faintness 19, 24, 110
Feeding difficulty (babies) 144–5
Feeling depressed 20–1, 22–3, 127, 129, 135
Feeling sad/tearful 20–1, 22–3
Feet, pain in 42, 43, 94, 97, 98, 99
Fever 12, 26, 27, 28, 29, 30, 31, 32, 33, 64, 78,
    79, 81, 104, 119, 135, 136, 138, 140, 142, 167
Flushing, skin 12, 40, 129, 135, 142, 167
Food cravings 127

G
Genitals, itching or soreness in 120, 133, 152
Glands, swollen 27, 28, 81
Groin
    itching 44
    pain 92, 112, 119
    swelling 28, 112
Gullet, pain in 107, 174
Gums, sore or bleeding 73, 74, 75

H
Hair
    excess 51
    flakes or specks in 49, 50, 151
    ingrowing 51
    loss 52
Headache 16, 20–1, 27, 28, 30, 32, 33, 78,
    81, 85, 86, 87, 104, 110, 111, 114, 116,
    127, 128, 135, 136
Head injury 157
Hearing, loss of 63, 64, 66, 68, 140
Heart rate, fast 24, 105
Heels, painful 97, 99
Hiccups 101
Hips, pain in 92
Hoarse voice 81, 82, 138
Hyperventilating 24

I, J, K
Incontinence 121, 129, 131, 139
Increased appetite 22–3
Irritability 17, 20–1, 127, 129, 141, 142
Itching 14, 35, 36, 38, 39, 41, 44, 48, 49, 50,
    95, 137, 158
Jaw, aching 79
Joint
    pain 27, 90, 91, 92, 93
    swollen 93, 95, 96, 160
Knee pain 93, 160

Symptom finder continued

L
Leg pain 88–9, 92, 94
Limb
  abnormal appearance of 161
  pain 160, 161
  swollen 160, 161
Lips
  cold sore on 70
  cracked or sore 69

M
Migraine 20–1, 86
Mood changes 20, 22, 25, 127, 129, 141
Mouth
  dry 72
  pain 71, 73, 75
Moving difficulty 87, 88–9, 90, 92, 93, 160, 161
Mucus
  in nose or throat 77
  in stools 111
Muscles
  aching 26, 30, 85, 87, 88–9, 104, 160
  cramps 94
  spasms or twitching 88–9, 94, 166, 167
  weakness 88–9

N, O
Nails
  bitten 54
  brittle 39, 53
  disfigured 39, 44, 53, 55
  loosened 39
Nausea 16, 24, 86, 106, 107, 109, 110, 111,
  113, 114, 115, 143, 165
Navel, swelling under 112
Neck
  stiff or sore 85, 87
  swollen 26
Nipples, painful or cracked 126
Nose
  bleeding 83
  blocked 77, 78, 79, 80
  itchy 80
  red 40
  runny 27, 29, 77, 78, 79, 80, 138
Numb areas 100

P, Q
Palpitations 24, 105
Panic 20–1, 24
Parasites 35, 50, 137
Passing out 19
Penis
  discharge from 120
  erection difficulty 122
  painful 120
Periods
  irregular 129
  painful 128
Personality change 20, 22, 25, 129
Phlegm 78, 104

Poor concentration 17, 18, 20–1, 22–3, 127, 129
Poor memory 20–1, 22–3, 25, 129
Pulse, abnormal 165

R
Rash
  blistering 32, 33
  itchy 32, 35, 36, 38, 44, 46–7, 113, 150
  nappy 152
  red 27, 29, 40, 44, 46–7, 113, 150, 152
Restlessness 86, 165

S
Sadness 20–1, 22–3
Scalp
  itchy 49, 50
  scaly 49, 151
Scrotum
  pain 119
  swelling 112, 119
Sensitivity to noise 86
Sex drive, loss of 22–3
Sexual difficulties 122, 123, 129, 134
Sexual intercourse, pain during 133, 134
Shaking/trembling 24
Shivering 12, 30, 135
Shoulder pain 85, 87, 90
Skin
  blue or grey 100, 159, 161, 164
  cold 100
  cracked 38, 41, 44
  dry 38, 39, 41, 46–7, 69, 95, 129, 164
  growths 43
  hard 42, 98
  hot 12, 135, 142, 160, 164
  itchy see Itching
  lumps or swellings 35, 36, 45, 59, 95,
    158, 164
  painful or tingling 33, 45, 46–7, 70, 100, 164
  red 36, 39, 40, 41, 46–7, 48, 49, 100, 158,
    159, 164
  scaly or flaky 38, 39, 41, 44, 48, 49, 151
  splinters 156
  spots or pimples 32, 33, 34, 37, 40, 150, 152
  white or pale 100, 110, 165
Sleeping
  difficulty 17, 18, 20–1, 22–3, 127, 146–7
  excessive 22–3
Smell, loss or alteration in sense of 77, 78, 86
Sneezing 78, 80, 138
Snoring 84
Sores
  face 34, 70
  mouth 71
  penis 120
Spots
  inside cheeks 29
  on skin 27, 29, 34, 37, 40, 46, 150, 152
Stools
  abnormal 111, 113, 115, 116, 136, 143
  difficulty passing 18, 111, 115, 127

Stress, signs of 17, 20–1, 24, 38, 111, 123, 127
Stuffed-up nose 77, 78, 79, 80
Swallowing difficulty 26, 81, 172
Sweating or clammy skin 12, 13, 24, 44, 109,
  110, 129, 165, 167
Swollen ankles 96
Swollen face 26, 159
Swollen glands 27, 28, 81
Swollen joints 93, 95, 96, 160

T
Talking, difficulty in 26
Taste, loss or alteration of 77, 78, 79, 86
Teeth
  aching 75, 79
  sensitive 75
Temperature, raised 12, 26, 27, 28, 29, 30, 31,
  32, 33, 64, 78, 79, 81, 104, 119, 135, 136,
  138, 140, 142, 167
Thirst 16, 165
Threadworms 137
Throat, sore 28, 30, 78, 81, 82
Tingling skin 33, 70, 100
Tiredness 15, 17, 18, 20–1, 22–3, 28, 30, 84
Toe, sore 42, 55, 98
Tonsils, swollen 81
Toothache 75
Tooth, knocked-out 76

U, V
Unconsciousness 159, 162, 164, 165, 166,
  167, 168, 169, 170–1
Urination
  difficulty 121
  painful 119, 120, 130, 133
  too frequent 121, 131, 139
Urine
  foul-smelling 130
  leakage of 121, 131, 139
Vagina
  discharge 132
  dryness 129
  itching 133
  pain 134
Veins, swollen 95, 117
Vision
  blurred 61
  disturbed 86
Voice, loss of 82
Vomiting 31, 86, 109, 110, 114, 116, 136, 141,
  143, 174
Vulva, itching 133, 137

W, X, Y, Z
Weakness 165
Weals 36
Weight gain 127
Wheezing 80, 103, 138, 159
Wind 106, 108, 111
Worms 137
Wounds 156, 157, 161, 162

COMMON CONDITIONS

This major part of the book features a wide range of common illnesses and disorders that can usually be treated successfully at home. The first section covers general symptoms, such as fever or tiredness, that are common to many illnesses, and is followed by the most prevalent infectious diseases. Conditions are then organized according to the parts of the body they affect, such as the chest and abdomen, or the eyes and ears. Specific problems affecting men, women, children, and babies are dealt with in their own sections.

GENERAL SYMPTOMS

Fever

In a fever, your body temperature is raised persistently above the normal level of 37°C (98.6°F). A fever is one way in which the body responds to infection, so it is most likely to result from a viral illness such as flu, or a throat, chest, or urinary infection. It can also be due to other diseases, to heatstroke, sunburn, or reactions to drugs. At first you feel warm; if your temperature goes on rising, you feel chilled and shivery, then as it drops you feel hot and flushed. You may become dehydrated if the fever persists.

> ## WARNING
> Get medical help straight away if:
> • Temperature is over 39.4°C (103°F)
> • You have a headache, sensitivity to light, stiff neck, and/or a rash
> • You are drowsy or confused
> • You have difficulty breathing

 ## See your doctor first

Arrange to see your doctor promptly if you feel weak and very unwell, and/or if you have a specific symptom with a fever, such as earache, a rash, or a cough with phlegm.

What you can do yourself

Use the following measures in conjunction with any treatment from your doctor.

• Rest; you don't have to stay in bed, but don't overexert yourself. Don't go to work.

 • Take a painkiller (see DRUG REMEDIES, right).

• Drink at least 8 glasses of water or weak fruit juice to help prevent dehydration. Aim to have 1 glass of fluid an hour. Avoid caffeinated drinks. Try soups and broths if you feel unable to eat.

• Keep cool, but avoid getting cold. Wear light, loose clothes. In hot weather, use an electric fan.

 • To check your temperature, use a digital thermometer (see PRACTICAL TECHNIQUE, right).

• If you are feeling shivery, don't try to warm yourself. Instead, cover yourself with a sheet or a light blanket.

• If you feel hot and sweaty, sponge your face with lukewarm water.

 ### DRUG REMEDIES

Painkillers such as paracetamol (see p.187) and ibuprofen (see p.184) will reduce fever and help to relieve headache and muscle aches. Start taking a painkiller as soon as you begin to feel feverish.

PRACTICAL TECHNIQUE

Checking your temperature Use a digital thermometer placed in your mouth or armpit, or an aural thermometer, the tip of which is inserted in the ear. Forehead temperature strips are not reliable.

Using a digital thermometer
Hold in place until it beeps, then read the temperature display.

Seek further medical advice

Arrange to see your doctor if:

• Your temperature keeps rising despite attempts to bring it down
• The fever has not subsided within 2 days and/or you have developed other symptoms

Excessive sweating

Almost everyone sweats more than usual when exercising or in hot weather, but some people generally sweat too much. Excessive sweating is common in adolescence but can continue throughout life. It can cause body odour and affect work and social relationships. People who sweat excessively are also more prone to fungal skin infections. Although some people are naturally susceptible to this problem, other factors, such as stress and anxiety, may have a significant role. Excessive sweating sometimes occurs in women around the time of the menopause, or as a feature of conditions such as an overactive thyroid gland.

➡ *See also* Athlete's foot and jock itch, p.44.

 ## See your doctor first

Make an appointment to see your doctor if:

- The sweating is prolonged or unusual
- You are losing weight

What you can do yourself

There are some useful home treatments that help to reduce sweating and body odour.

- Bathe or shower at least once daily in warm (but not hot) water. Dry yourself thoroughly afterwards.

- Use an antiperspirant or an antiperspirant combined with a deodorant. If an ordinary product does not work, try a stronger preparation containing aluminium chloride (*see* DRUG REMEDIES, right).

- Wear clean underwear and clothes every day. Choose natural fabrics, such as cotton, particularly next to your skin. Avoid tight clothes.

- If your feet get sweaty, wear leather shoes and cotton socks, and change both regularly. Go barefoot or wear sandals whenever possible.

- Drink at least 8 glasses of water a day, to replace lost body fluids. Cut down on alcohol and drinks containing caffeine, particularly hot drinks.

- Avoid spicy foods, which are likely to make you sweat, and onions and garlic, because of the odour.

- If you sweat when you are anxious, try practical techniques that reduce stress (*see* pp.20–21).

- If you are overweight, try to lose some weight.

DRUG REMEDIES

Antiperspirants and deodorants
Antiperspirants block the pores that produce sweat, while deodorants attack the skin bacteria that cause body odour. Many products contain a combination of the two. Apply them daily after washing. If you develop skin irritation, use a hypoallergenic product. Absorbent, deodorizing foot powders are available for feet.

Aluminium chloride preparations
(*see* p.177) treat severe sweating from the armpits, hands, or feet. These are usually roll-ons that are applied to dry skin each night and washed off the next day. Use the product less often as sweating decreases. Don't use it on broken or irritated skin, close to the eyes or lips, or if you have shaved or removed hair from the skin in the previous 12 hours.

Using aluminium chloride
Wash thoroughly and make sure that your skin is completely dry before you apply the antiperspirant.

 ## Seek further medical advice

Arrange to see your doctor if:

- You are still troubled by excessive sweating or body odour after following the advice described here
- You have any other symptoms associated with the excessive sweating

Itching

Itching is often a minor problem, but continual scratching may damage your skin and make the problem worse. A small area of itching may be caused by an insect bite or occur with a rash as a reaction to plants, metals, chemicals, or cosmetics. Larger areas may be due to dry skin, heat rash, hives, infections such as ringworm or scabies, or skin diseases such as eczema and psoriasis. Itching all over the body can be due to disorders such as diabetes, liver problems, or drug reactions. Stress and anxiety may cause or aggravate itching.

 See also Scabies, p.35; Hives, p.36; Eczema, p.38; Psoriasis, p.39; Dry skin, p.41; Athlete's foot and jock itch, p.44; Heat rash, p.46; Ringworm, p.48; Genital irritation, p.133; Insect bites and stings, p.158.

 ### See your doctor first

Consult your doctor if you think itching may be caused by a prescribed medicine.

What you can do yourself

There are several measures that you can take to help relieve itching.

- Try to resist scratching, and keep your fingernails short to limit any damage.

- Apply a cold compress. Soak a clean face cloth in cold water, wring it out, then place it on the itchy area. Repeat as necessary.

 • Apply a soothing preparation such as calamine lotion or crotamiton cream (*see* DRUG REMEDIES, right).

• Try a mild hydrocortisone cream (*see* DRUG REMEDIES, right) for a localized area of red, itchy skin caused by an irritant, such as a cleaning product or metal jewellery. The cream is also helpful for insect bites and stings.

 • Take antihistamine tablets to relieve itching that keeps you awake at night (*see* DRUG REMEDIES, right). Antihistamine cream can be used to relieve insect bites and stings.

- Moisturize and protect dry skin (*see* p.41).

- If stress aggravates itching, try some deep breathing exercises and muscle relaxation techniques (*see* PRACTICAL TECHNIQUES, pp.20–21).

- If possible, avoid hot or humid environments.

- Wear loose-fitting clothes made from natural fibres, but avoid wearing wool next to your skin.

 ### DRUG REMEDIES

Calamine lotion (*see* p.179) has a cooling effect. Apply it to itchy areas as often as needed.

Crotamiton preparations (*see* p.180) help to soothe irritated skin and reduce itching.

Hydrocortisone cream (*see* p.184) reduces itching and redness and is useful for treating allergic skin reactions and insect stings. Don't use it on children under 10 without medical advice.

Sedating antihistamines (*see* p.178) such as chlorphenamine are taken orally to relieve itching. They will also help you to sleep. Use a cream for itchy insect bites and stings.

 ### PREVENTION

Avoiding triggers for itching Once itching is under control, try to identify what causes it or makes it worse, if this isn't already obvious.

- Keep a diary, noting when you feel itchy and which products you use on your skin or clothing. If you suspect itching is due to a skin product, switch to a mild, unperfumed brand. If the cause is a washing powder, use a non-biological one and an extra rinse.

Seek further medical advice

Arrange to see your doctor if:

- Itching does not subside after about a week
- You develop other symptoms, such as jaundice or weight loss

Tiredness

Everyone feels tired after physical exertion or long periods of hard work. A good night's sleep usually solves the problem, but sometimes tiredness seems to drag on for days, and can interfere with your daily activities. The most obvious cause is difficulty in sleeping, but you may also feel tired if you are stressed or a bit low, or if you've recently suffered an upset such as a bereavement. An unhealthy diet and lack of exercise are common contributory factors. Viral illnesses such as glandular fever and flu can leave you tired for weeks afterwards. Sometimes, persistent tiredness is due to an underlying condition such as anaemia or a thyroid problem.

 See also Difficulty sleeping, p.17; Stress, pp.20–21; Feeling depressed, pp.22–23.

See your doctor first

Make an appointment to see your doctor if:

- Tiredness is persistent and sleep doesn't help
- You often feel tired for no apparent reason

What you can do yourself

If you're feeling tired all the time, try the following adjustments to help you get your energy back.

- Even when you're very busy, get enough sleep each night. Overdoing things, then trying to catch up on your rest at the weekends, will throw out your sleep routine and leave you even more tired.

- Never miss breakfast. Include fresh vegetables, fruit, cereals, and wholemeal bread, pasta, and rice in your diet. Cut down on fatty foods such as cheese, eggs, and red meat, and on sugar and salt.

- Check that you are not overweight or too thin. If you need to lose or gain weight, do so gradually.

- Try to spend time each day in fresh air. Exercise regularly, particularly if you have a sedentary job.

- If you are sleepy during the day or while driving, try a "power nap" (*see* PRACTICAL TECHNIQUE, right).

- If you have had a viral illness, such as glandular fever or flu, it may be several weeks before you're back to normal. Take time off to recover and take things easy when you return to work or school.

- If stress is contributing to "burn out", make more time for leisure activities. Try some deep breathing and muscle relaxation exercises (*see* PRACTICAL TECHNIQUES, pp.20–21).

PRACTICAL TECHNIQUE

Power napping If you find yourself nodding off during the day or you feel drowsy while driving, a brief nap may help you to function better.

- An ideal nap lasts about 10–15 minutes, but even a 5-minute sleep will leave you brighter and sharper afterwards. Sleeping for more than 15 minutes helps, but you may feel groggy afterwards. More than 30 minutes may affect your ability to sleep at night.
- Take a daily nap at the same time each day so your body gets used to the routine. Use an alarm clock or watch if you are worried about sleeping for too long.
- Don't nap late in the day or fall asleep in front of the TV in the evening, and don't use naps to catch up on sleep if you are having difficulty sleeping.

Timed nap
Set a watch or clock to wake you from your nap after about 15 minutes.

Seek further medical advice

Arrange to see your doctor if:

- You still feel tired after trying these measures for 2–3 weeks, or you develop other symptoms

Hangover

A hangover is usually the result of drinking too much alcohol, but some people have symptoms after just a small amount of alcohol. The cause is a combination of the dehydrating effects of alcohol and adverse reactions to chemical additives in drinks, particularly dark-coloured drinks such as red wine, port, brandy, and sherry. You may have a headache, nausea, dizziness, a dry mouth, and a raging thirst, which may disturb your sleep at night. Most people recover rapidly with some self-help measures.

 See also Headache, p.85; Nausea and vomiting, p.109.

What you can do yourself

If you know you have drunk too much, take the following steps immediately to minimize a hangover. Most symptoms clear up within 24 hours.

- Drink plenty of non-alcoholic fluids before going to bed and the next morning to reduce dehydration. Have a glass of water by your bed, and take sips if you wake up in the night. Fruit juices, which contain the natural sugar fructose, are particularly helpful (*see* NATURAL REMEDIES, right). Don't drink tea or coffee because they irritate the stomach and increase dehydration.

- Eat if you can. Even a banana will help to boost low blood sugar levels.

- Take a painkiller to help prevent or relieve a headache (*see* DRUG REMEDIES, right).

- An antacid will help to reduce nausea, or try a hangover remedy (*see* DRUG REMEDIES, right).

- Don't drink more alcohol to reduce your symptoms; this will only prolong the hangover.

- Rest until you begin to feel better.

- Don't drive. Alcohol remains in the bloodstream for long periods, so you may still be unsafe to drive the day after you have been drinking.

Seek medical advice

Arrange to see your doctor if:

- You have regular hangovers and are finding it hard to reduce your drinking
- You feel the need to drink alcohol first thing in the morning

NATURAL REMEDIES

Fructose is a natural sugar that can help the body to burn up alcohol faster. Plenty of fruit, juices, and honey will help you to recover from a hangover.

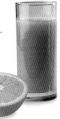

Source of fructose
Eat an orange or drink some freshly-squeezed juice to speed recovery.

DRUG REMEDIES

Painkillers such as ibuprofen (*see* p.184) or paracetamol (*see* p.187) will help relieve a headache. Taking ibuprofen before you go to sleep may actually prevent some of the symptoms of a hangover (although it may worsen any stomach irritation).

Antacids (*see* p.177) are taken to relieve nausea and indigestion. They are available as hard or chewy tablets, fizzy drinks, or soothing liquids.

Hangover remedies (*see* p.183) include painkillers, vitamins, antacids, and glucose, and can help to relieve the full range of hangover symptoms.

PREVENTION

Avoiding a hangover If you know you are going to drink alcohol, try the following steps.

- Eat a meal before you start drinking.
- Alternate between alcoholic and soft drinks.

Difficulty sleeping

Many people have difficulty sleeping, either because they find it hard to get to sleep at night or because they wake early and cannot get back to sleep. Adults need 7–8 hours of sleep, on average, but people need less as they get older, and elderly people may need as little as 5–6 hours. An occasional sleepless night won't do you any harm, although you may feel tired the next day. More persistent sleep disturbances are often due to stress, anxiety, or depression and may leave you continually tired, irritable, and unable to concentrate. Physical symptoms such as pain, breathing problems, and hot flushes, and some medicines, can also disturb sleep.

 See also Stress, pp.20–21; **Feeling depressed**, pp.22–23.

 ## See your doctor first

Make an appointment to see your doctor if:

- You feel depressed
- Physical symptoms are preventing sleep

What you can do yourself

There are several things you can try to make it easier to get a good night's sleep.

- Go to bed and get up at the same times each day. Even if you are tired, don't take naps during the day.

- Don't eat a heavy or rich meal less than 3 hours before you go to bed. Avoid coffee, tea, cola, alcohol, and smoking. If you are hungry, eat a biscuit or a banana. Drink a glass of warm milk half an hour before bedtime.

 - Use practical measures to help you get over your sleep difficulties (*see* PRACTICAL TIPS, right).

 - Try a herbal remedy that promotes sleep (*see* NATURAL REMEDIES, right).

 - If you're feeling tense, practise relaxation exercises (*see* pp.20–21) shortly before bedtime. Soak in a warm bath. Lavender oil (*see* NATURAL REMEDIES, right) may be helpful.

 - Taking a sedative antihistamine may relieve a temporary sleep problem (*see* DRUG REMEDIES, right).

Seek further medical advice

Arrange to see your doctor if you still cannot sleep after trying the measures given above.

PRACTICAL TIPS

Managing sleeplessness Try these tips, and keep using them until they begin to work.

- Stop working at least an hour before bedtime and read a book or listen to relaxing music. Keep your bedroom quiet, dark, and not too hot or cold.
- If you can't fall asleep within 30 minutes, get up, go into another room, and read. Don't watch TV.
- If your head is buzzing with tasks for the next day, keep a notepad by your bed and jot them down.

NATURAL REMEDIES

Herbal sleeping remedies (*see* p.183) Syrup or tablets containing valerian, passionflower, or hops may help to promote restful sleep.

Lavender oil (*see* p.184) is a traditional sleep remedy. Try inhaling it, or adding it to a warm bath before bedtime.

Using lavender
Try putting a bag of dried lavender or some drops of lavender oil on a tissue inside your pillowcase.

DRUG REMEDIES

Sedative antihistamines (*see* p.178) are useful for treating short-term insomnia.

Jet lag

Jet lag is a collection of symptoms that occur while your body clock adjusts to a new time zone when you travel. Until you get used to the local time, you may feel disoriented and tired during the day and have difficulty sleeping at the new night-time. You may also experience poor concentration, loss of appetite, and diarrhoea or constipation. Most people begin to feel the effects of jet lag only after crossing three or more time zones. Travelling from east to west (for example, from London to New York) extends the day and is usually easier on the body than travelling from west to east, which shortens the day. People tend to become more susceptible to the effects of jet lag as they get older.

What you can do yourself

Although jet lag usually lasts no more than a few days, use these tips to reduce its effects and adjust quickly to the new time zone.

- If possible, fly during the day. You are less likely to feel jet lag if you arrive at your destination in the evening and then stay awake until bedtime.

- Get plenty of rest before you depart: at least 8 hours' sleep a night in the week before you travel.

 • Start adjusting to the new time zone when you begin your journey (*see* PRACTICAL TIPS, right).

- Drink plenty of water or fruit juice before and during the flight to prevent dehydration, and avoid alcohol, coffee, or cola drinks. Eat light meals and avoid fatty or salty foods.

- As soon as you arrive at your destination, adopt the local eating, waking, and sleeping times. Take a walk in daylight to help your body clock adjust.

- Avoid alcohol or caffeinated drinks within 3 hours of bedtime as they will make sleep more difficult.

- Jet lag can affect judgement and concentration, so do not drive until you have adapted to local time.

 • If you travel frequently, try using antihistamine tablets to relieve temporary sleep disturbances (*see* DRUG REMEDIES, right). Alternatively, ask your doctor for a short-acting prescription sleeping pill.

- If you are spending less than 2 days in a new time zone, you may be better off getting up, eating, and sleeping according to your home time.

- Seek your doctor's advice before travelling if you have to take prescribed medicines, such as insulin or the contraceptive pill, at specific times of the day.

PRACTICAL TIPS

Adjusting to time zones Get used to the new time zone by setting your watch to your destination time as soon as you board the plane. If possible, plan your meals and sleep times around this time during the flight.

- If you need to sleep on the flight, listen to soft music, use earplugs, wear eyeshades, and use a neck pillow.
- If you need to stay awake, keep active: get up and walk around the plane every hour, talk to your neighbour, read, or watch the in-flight entertainment.

DRUG REMEDIES

Sedative antihistamines (*see* p.178) cause drowsiness and can be used for a few days to help you re-establish your normal sleeping pattern. These medications are not addictive. Ask your pharmacist for advice on a suitable type.

✚ Seek medical advice

Arrange to see your doctor if:

- You are still experiencing symptoms of jet lag 2 weeks after travelling

Feeling dizzy or faint

Dizzy spells and feeling faint are common problems. Causes include low blood sugar, drinking too much alcohol, or simply getting up too quickly. Feeling faint may also be due to emotional shock or panic, or may occur in pregnancy. An occasional attack is rarely a cause for concern, but sometimes the problem is due to an underlying condition or to certain drugs.

 See also Panic attacks, p.24.

> **WARNING**
>
> Seek immediate medical help if you are dizzy or faint and have:
> - Diabetes
> - Chest pain or palpitations
> - Weakness in your arms or legs, slurred speech, or blurred vision

 ## See your doctor first

Make an appointment to see your doctor if:

- You are taking a prescribed medicine that may be causing the problem, such as drugs for high blood pressure or tranquillizers

What you can do yourself

There are several things you can do to help you get over a faint or dizzy spell quickly.

- Keep your head down on your knees or your feet raised and try to control your breathing (*see* PRACTICAL TECHNIQUE, right).

- If it has been several hours since you last ate, eat or drink a sugary snack (not something containing artificial sweeteners).

- Don't drink caffeinated drinks such as coffee, tea, or cola, or alcohol, and don't smoke, as all of these can make your symptoms worse.

- Don't try to drive or operate machinery until you are completely recovered.

 ## Seek further medical advice

Arrange to see your doctor if:

- You do not recover promptly from an episode of dizziness or feeling faint
- You have repeated episodes of feeling faint or dizzy, or you develop any other symptoms

PRACTICAL TECHNIQUE

Recovery measures If you feel faint or dizzy, sit down and put your head on your knees. Alternatively, lie down and raise your legs on a chair or cushion. Try to keep calm, because fast breathing (hyperventilating) and anxiety can make symptoms worse. Breathe slowly and deeply. Open a window or go out into fresh air if you feel steady on your feet.

Helping blood flow
Lean forward and put your head down to improve the blood flow to your brain.

PREVENTION

Avoiding dizzy spells Combine these steps with any treatment from your doctor to help prevent further attacks.

- Avoid hot and stuffy environments. Have a window open, or go out into fresh air from time to time.
- Don't get up suddenly after lying down or sitting.
- Drink at least 6–8 glasses of water a day.
- Eat regularly. Have healthy snacks, such as fruit, between meals to keep your blood sugar level steady.
- Try to avoid straining on the toilet, as this can cause a drop in blood pressure and make you feel faint.
- If you are pregnant, don't stand for long periods or lie flat on your back.

Stress

When you are under stress, your muscles tighten, your heart beats faster, your breathing becomes rapid and shallow, and your brain becomes more alert. In small doses, stress can improve your performance in situations such as sport or work, but if excessive or prolonged it can harm your health. You may suffer poor appetite, headaches, migraine, difficulty sleeping, and increased susceptibility to infections. You may also feel anxious, irritable, unable to concentrate, tired, sad, or depressed. Stress tends to build up when the normal pressures of life become too much for you, or may be triggered by an upsetting event such as a bereavement.

 See also Tiredness, p.15; Difficulty sleeping, p.17; Feeling depressed, pp.22–23; Panic attacks, p.24.

What you can do yourself

People react differently to stress depending on their personality and the support they have around them. Although you can't always control difficult events in your life, you can adapt the way in which you react to everyday stresses and learn how to avoid some of them.

● Get adequate sleep; if you are tired you are more likely to feel stressed.

● Eat regularly to keep your energy levels constant during the day. Never miss breakfast. Include fresh fruit, cereal, wholemeal bread, pasta, and rice in your diet. Cut down on foods such as cheese, eggs, red meat, and butter that are high in fat. Reduce your intake of sugar and salt.

● Cut down or cut out caffeine by limiting your intake of coffee, tea, cola, and chocolate.

● Take regular exercise, especially if you have a sedentary job. Exercise produces "feel-good" chemicals in the brain that increase your sense of wellbeing. Try 15–30 minutes of brisk walking, or go swimming or cycling.

● Set aside a regular time each day specifically for relaxation: do not wait until you feel exhausted. Go for a regular walk; listen to music; or try meditation or yoga.

● Imagine that you are in a place where you feel warm, relaxed, and comfortable, such as lying on a sunny beach. Try to imagine all the colours, sounds, smells, and feelings.

 ● Practise deep, controlled breathing with exercises that can be used whenever you feel tense (*see* PRACTICAL TECHNIQUE, right).

PRACTICAL TECHNIQUE

Deep breathing This exercise helps to calm your body and mind. Deep breathing using the diaphragm and abdominal muscles is the basis of most relaxation methods. Find a place where you won't be interrupted, take the phone off the hook and/or switch off your mobile phone, and practise these exercises for 10–20 minutes each day.

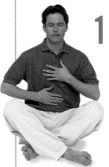

1 *Wear loose clothing and sit or lie in a comfortable position. Place one hand on your chest and the other on your abdomen. Breathe in slowly through your nose, hold your breath for a moment, then breathe out slowly. Try to breathe using your abdominal muscles so the lower hand moves more than the upper one.*

2 *Once you know that you are breathing from your abdomen, place your hands just below your ribs. Feel your hands move as your abdomen rises and falls. When you feel more relaxed, let your hands drop down by your sides and simply enjoy the relaxation.*

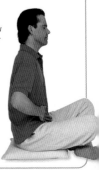

What you can do yourself *continued...*

- When you are in the middle of a stressful situation, try to have a few minutes alone. Go for a brisk walk or sit somewhere quiet to help you relax.

- If your muscles have become tense, try to relax them at will (*see* PRACTICAL TECHNIQUE, right).

- Try to control self-criticism. To counteract it, remind yourself of your good points and the successes you have had in the past.

- Don't bottle up your worries; it usually helps to share problems with family members and friends.

- Don't try a short-term "fix" by turning to alcohol or illicit drugs. In the long term they will only add to your problems.

Seek medical advice

Arrange to see your doctor if:

- You feel unable to cope with stress
- You feel depressed

PREVENTION

Limiting stress If you have a great deal of stress, the following steps will help you identify the causes, deal with them and feel healthier as a result.

- Over 2–3 weeks, make a note of the situations in which you felt under stress and whether stress made you perform better or worse than normal. Think about how you might have responded differently to feel more in control. Ask people close to you how they react in similar situations.
- Accept that there are some things you can't control, such as traffic hold-ups on the way to work.
- Organize and prioritize your time. Do what is important first. Anticipate deadlines and reduce your other commitments around these times.
- Identify tasks and break them into smaller sections if they seem too big to cope with all at once. Use a checklist and tick off tasks as you complete them.
- Have realistic expectations. Don't commit yourself to tasks that you feel unable to do or don't want to do; delegate when you are able to do so. Don't feel demoralized or guilty if things go wrong.
- Take regular breaks through the day, even if it is only to look out of the window. Have lunch breaks.

PRACTICAL TECHNIQUE

Relaxing muscles Learn to recognize when your muscles are tense, as this will help you to control stress reactions. This exercise will enable you to relax problem areas consciously. If time is short, it may help to use the exercise on just one group of muscles, such as your shoulders. Keep your eyes closed throughout, and breathe slowly using your abdominal muscles (*see* opposite page).

1 To prepare for the exercise, be aware of how your muscles feel in their relaxed state and when they are tense. Try to imagine the tension fading away as you relax each muscle.

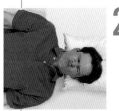

2 Yawn, then relax. Clench your jaw, and release. Frown, scrunch up your eyes and nose, then let go. Raise your eyebrows, then relax all the muscles in your face.

3 Lift your shoulders up to your ears. Hold for a few seconds, then lower again. Repeat 2–3 times. To free the neck muscles, rock your head gently from side to side.

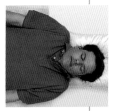

4 Tense and relax your stomach muscles, then each buttock in turn. Clench and release your right fist, then all the muscles in your arm. Repeat the process with your left arm.

5 Tense the muscles in your right foot, hold for a few seconds, then release. Tense and release the calf, then the thigh muscles. Repeat the process with the left foot and leg.

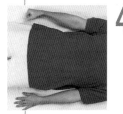

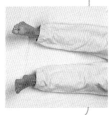

Feeling depressed

Most people have occasional low moods, but if you are depressed they become persistent. You may feel tearful and low, particularly in the morning; lack energy and confidence; and find it hard to concentrate or make decisions. Sleep problems and loss of sex drive and appetite are common. Depression is often a reaction to a life event such as bereavement, or it may have no obvious cause. Lack of sunlight in winter makes some people feel sad, and 1 woman in 10 has depression after childbirth.

 See also Stress, pp.20–21.

> **WARNING**
>
> Seek immediate medical help if:
> - You are having suicidal thoughts
> - You have recently had a baby and are having thoughts of harming yourself or your child

✚ See your doctor first

Make an appointment to see your doctor if you have feelings of depression that last longer than a week.

What you can do yourself

There are several lifestyle changes and home treatments that can help you through a short period of feeling low. They will also support treatment given by your doctor.

- When you are depressed, even simple tasks may seem difficult. Set a small, achievable, pleasant goal for yourself each day, such as taking a walk around the block or having a special breakfast. Adopt the same approach if you feel you have an overwhelming list of problems. Tackle only one problem at a time; if necessary, break it down into smaller, achievable goals and work through them.

- If you have occasional sad or negative thoughts, distract yourself by listening to the radio or watching TV, which require little concentration.

- Try to avoid extra stress. If possible, postpone or delegate important decisions. Look rationally at the work you have to do; focus on essential tasks and sideline less important ones.

- Don't bottle things up. You may find it a relief to share your feelings and emotions with sympathetic relatives or close friends. Talking about problems is not a sign of weakness.

NATURAL REMEDIES

St John's wort (*see* p.189) is a popular herbal remedy for mild depression. Taken as a tablet once a day, it appears to be as effective as some prescription antidepressants. Like prescribed drugs, it can take some time to work.

CAUTION: Check with your doctor before taking St John's wort. Don't use it if you are already taking prescribed antidepressants or the contraceptive pill.

Essential fatty acids (*see* p.181), or EFAs, are obtained from foods and play an important part in forming healthy cells and nerve tissue. A group called omega-3 EFAs may also help to regulate hormones and brain chemicals that control mood, and can help to reduce symptoms of depression. You can boost levels of these EFAs by eating olive oil, walnuts, and oily fish, such as salmon and mackerel.

Boosting omega-3 EFAs
Make sure your diet includes 2 or 3 portions a week of oily fish, such as grilled mackerel.

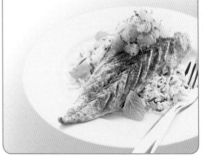

What you can do yourself *continued...*

- Try to eat regularly, even though you may not feel like it. Choose foods that you enjoy, but make sure you include plenty of vegetables, fruit, bread, pasta, rice, and potatoes. Have small portions if you don't feel like eating large meals.

- Exercise helps you relax, improves sleep, and may reduce depression by releasing chemicals in the brain that improve mood. Just going for a walk or doing some gardening is beneficial. Everybody should be capable of taking some exercise, but if you have a medical condition (such as arthritis or a heart problem), check with your doctor first.

- Try the natural remedy St John's wort to relieve low moods (*see* NATURAL REMEDIES, left).

- Include foods such as oily fish and olive oil in your diet to boost your levels of essential fatty acids, or EFAs (*see* NATURAL REMEDIES, left). These substances may help to combat depression.

- Cut down or stop drinking alcohol. Although it may appear to offer a "quick fix", alcohol can contribute to depression and also affects your physical health.

- Stop using any recreational drugs, such as cannabis or ecstasy; they can have long-term effects that contribute to depression.

- If your sleep is disturbed, try reducing your caffeine intake, and avoid sleeping in the day (*see* DIFFICULTY SLEEPING, p.17).

- If you regularly feel tense and find it difficult to unwind, try practising deep breathing exercises and muscle relaxation methods (*see* PRACTICAL TECHNIQUES, pp.20–21).

- If possible, try to identify the cause of your depression. Defining your problem may help you to stop feeling guilty about your feelings and, with time, you may become able to deal with the underlying difficulty.

- If you are regularly depressed in the winter months (a condition known as seasonal affective disorder, or SAD) you may benefit from light treatment (*see* PRACTICAL TIPS, right).

PRACTICAL TIPS

Coping with SAD Symptoms of seasonal affective disorder usually develop as the days get shorter in autumn. You may feel sad, low, and tired, want to sleep more than you normally do, and have cravings for starchy or sugary foods. Increased exposure to natural light is thought to help SAD sufferers, so try the following tips.

- Try to get outdoors as much as possible on winter days. Even on dull, cloudy days you will benefit from exposure to natural light.
- Arrange work and home conditions so that you are exposed to as much natural light as possible. Work by a window if you can. Trim back trees and bushes around your home to let in light.
- If possible, treat yourself to a short winter break in a sunny country.
- Some people find light therapy helpful. This is usually given using a special light box that emits a very bright light. Other devices simulate a natural dawn in the morning. Light boxes are usually expensive, so discuss what might be of value with your doctor before you invest in equipment.

Using light therapy
You can carry out normal activities, such as reading, working, or eating, while staying close to the light box.

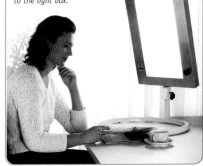

 ## Seek further medical advice

Arrange to see your doctor if:

- **Your depression is becoming more severe and/or lasts longer than 2 weeks**
- **You are taking prescribed antidepressant drugs and they are not having an effect within the timespan suggested by your doctor**

Panic attacks

Panic attacks are episodes of intense fear with unpleasant physical symptoms that usually occur without any outside threat being present. You may be short of breath or breathe rapidly (hyperventilate) and suffer from sweating, dizziness, nausea, numbness, chest pains, or palpitations. Attacks may be linked to anxiety, stress, depression, a phobia (such as fear of flying), or to taking stimulants or drugs, but symptoms can develop for no apparent reason. Although the attacks usually pass quickly, fear of having them can interfere with normal life.

See also Stress, pp.20–21; Feeling depressed, pp.22–23; Palpitations, p.105.

 ## See your doctor first

Make an appointment to see your doctor to check that your symptoms aren't due to a more serious illness such as heart disease.

What you can do yourself

Take the following steps to calm yourself quickly and help you cope with future attacks.

● If you are hyperventilating, try rebreathing into a bag (*see* PRACTICAL TECHNIQUE, right).

● When you feel symptoms developing, focus steadily on something happening near to you or on what someone else is saying, rather than concentrating on your own feelings. Remind yourself that, although your symptoms are unpleasant, they cannot harm you and will pass.

● Try not to avoid situations in which you are prone to attacks. If you start to confront them, your symptoms should begin to fade and you will begin to regain your confidence.

 ### PRACTICAL TECHNIQUE

Rebreathing into a paper bag
Rapid breathing during a panic attack lowers carbon dioxide levels in your blood, making you feel dizzy and faint. Rebreathing from a paper bag, held loosely over your mouth and nose, will help to restore carbon dioxide levels. Cup your hands over your mouth and nose if you don't have a bag.

Using a paper bag
Breathe in and out into the bag about 10 times, then breathe normally for 15 seconds. Continue until your breathing slows down.

 ## Seek further medical advice

Arrange to see your doctor if:

● The above measures do not help
● Your panic attacks are becoming more frequent and/or are interfering with your life

 ### PREVENTION

Preventing panic attacks The following lifestyle changes and techniques can help to prevent or at least minimize panic attacks.

● Practise deep breathing and muscle relaxation exercises (*see* PRACTICAL TECHNIQUES, pp.20–21) and use them whenever an attack is about to begin.
● Too much caffeine may trigger attacks, so reduce your intake of caffeinated drinks. Cut down on alcohol and smoking and don't take recreational drugs.
● Eat regular meals to keep your sugar levels stable and prevent symptoms such as lightheadedness.
● Exercise regularly to boost your general wellbeing.

Poor memory

Most people suffer from occasional forgetfulness, especially in later life when slower brain processing may make it harder for them to store and remember information. However, absentmindedness is not an inevitable part of aging, nor is it confined to the elderly. Poor memory can also be due to lack of sleep; an underlying condition such as depression; stress; a thyroid disorder; excessive use of alcohol; or prescribed or recreational drugs. In most cases, memory improves again when the underlying problem is treated. There are also techniques that help to protect and sharpen memory skills at any age. When memory deterioration occurs with symptoms such as confusion, intellectual decline, and a change in personality, it may be a sign of dementia.

 ## See your doctor first

Make an appointment to see your doctor if:

- Your memory is deteriorating
- You are taking medication such as sleeping tablets that may be affecting your memory

What you can do yourself

There are no instant cures for forgetfulness, but the following techniques and lifestyle changes can help preserve and improve your memory.

- Get a good night's sleep, take regular exercise, and include plenty of fresh fruits (especially citrus fruits), green leafy vegetables, nuts, olives, granary bread, and cereals in your diet.

- Try not to worry about your memory failures; anxiety and lack of confidence will only make them worse. Work out why you forgot something and organize yourself so it is less likely to happen again.

 - Try techniques to improve your memory (*see* PRACTICAL TECHNIQUES, right). Exercise your brain with crosswords and word games. Read a book or newspaper rather than watch TV passively.

- Note tasks and events on a calendar and in a diary that you keep with you at all times. Be orderly: keep essential articles in their own place, such as keys and glasses by the front door. Have fixed days and times for important tasks.

- Don't drink to excess or take recreational drugs such as cannabis and ecstasy. However, drinking 1–2 units of alcohol every day (a glass of wine is 1 unit) may help to reduce the risk of dementia.

- Have your vision and hearing checked regularly.

 ### PRACTICAL TECHNIQUES

Memory aids Most of the following techniques use visualization and repetition, which help to store information in memory.

- Pay attention, particularly in situations where you feel excited or under stress. Ask people to repeat information that doesn't register immediately. Then repeat it in your own words. Note landmarks along your route in unfamiliar surroundings such as a large building or driving through a new town.
- If you tend to forget a person's name moments after you are introduced, repeat the name back, then try to make a picture from it incorporating the person in front of you. For example, visualize Glenda Fisher in a leafy glen, fishing by a stream.
- To remember a list, use a set of locations in your home and put an item from the list in each one. Make the mental images incongruous and exaggerated. For example, to remember a shopping list you could visualize a huge block of butter melting on your bed; a loaf of bread baking in the fireplace; or a giant teabag in the washbasin. To recall the list in the supermarket, visualize walking through your home and finding each item in its strange location.
- Exercise your memory. Keep track of your money by remembering how and where you spent it since you last went to the bank. Alternatively, try to recall the main points of a recent conversation with a friend.

 ## Seek further medical advice

Arrange to see your doctor if:

- Your memory is continuing to decline and/or you are finding it difficult to cope

INFECTIOUS DISEASES

Mumps

Mumps is a viral infection that was common in children before routine immunization. The incubation period is 2–3 weeks. The illness usually starts with a fever, headache, and muscle aches. These are usually followed by swelling on one or both sides of the face and neck of the parotid salivary glands, which are just in front of and below the ears. Talking, eating, and drinking may be painful. Mumps is usually mild in children, but teenagers and adults may develop potentially serious complications.

> ### WARNING
>
> Contact your doctor urgently if any of the following develop:
> - Severe headache and dislike of bright light
> - Vomiting, seizures, or excessive drowsiness

 ## See your doctor first

Make an appointment to see your doctor to confirm mumps and check for complications.

What you can do yourself

There is no specific treatment for mumps, but you can make yourself or your child more comfortable.

- Rest until symptoms begin to ease.

- A warm compress, such as a face flannel soaked in warm water, applied to the side of the face, can help to relieve pain in swollen glands.

- Drink plenty of fluids, but avoid acidic fruit juices because they stimulate saliva and may make the enlarged glands more painful. Use a straw if opening the mouth is painful.

- Have soups, yoghurts and other soft, bland foods that are easy to swallow.

 - A painkiller will help reduce fever and relieve aches and pains (*see* DRUG REMEDIES, right).

- If mumps affects the testicles, stay in bed and wear supportive clothing, such as two pairs of close-fitting underpants, until symptoms ease.

- If there are no complications, a child can usually go back to school, or an adult can return to work, 5 days after the onset of swollen glands. However, full recovery can take 1–2 weeks.

 ### DRUG REMEDIES

Painkillers will bring down a fever and relieve muscle aches and the pain of swollen glands.

- For a child, give paracetamol (*see* p.187). This drug is available in a variety of forms, such as liquid medicine, soluble tablets, or melt-in-the-mouth tablets. Alternatively, you can give liquid ibuprofen (*see* p.184). Your pharmacist will advise you which is most suitable for your child.
- Adults can take paracetamol (*see* p.187) or ibuprofen (*see* p.184).

 ### PREVENTION

Immunization to protect against mumps is given as part of the MMR (measles, mumps, rubella) vaccine. Make sure your child is immunized.

 ## Seek further medical advice

Arrange to see your doctor if you or your child develops:

- Pain in the abdomen or chest
- Swelling and pain in the testicles

Rubella

Rubella (German measles) is a contagious viral illness that is now uncommon due to immunization. Usually, it causes little more than a mild red rash that spreads from the face to the body. Often there are no symptoms. A child may start with a mild fever, swollen glands, and a runny nose 2–3 weeks after contact with the infection. Adults may also have a headache and joint pain. The main risk of rubella is that it can harm the fetus if a woman contracts the virus in pregnancy, particularly in the early months.

WARNING

Contact your doctor immediately if:
- You are pregnant and suspect you may have been in contact with someone who has rubella

See your doctor first

Arrange to see your doctor if you suspect that you have rubella. Check when to attend the surgery, because of the risk of infecting a woman who is pregnant.

What you can do yourself

When there are symptoms, they are often so mild they need little or no treatment. The rash does not itch and disappears within a few days.

- Take a painkiller to reduce fever and relieve headache and joint pain (see DRUG REMEDIES, right).

- Drink plenty of fluids to prevent dehydration.

- As soon as you think that you have rubella, avoid contact with anyone who might be pregnant. Rubella is infectious for about 7 days before the rash develops and for about 5 days afterwards.

Seek further medical advice

Arrange to see your doctor if you develop:

- Headache or drowsiness
- Joint pain or sore eyes

DRUG REMEDIES

Painkillers will help bring down a fever and relieve headache and joint pain.

- For a child, give paracetamol (see p.187) or ibuprofen (see p.184), which are available in various forms. Ask your pharmacist for advice.
- Adults can take paracetamol (see p.187) or ibuprofen (see p.184).

PREVENTION

Immunization against rubella is given as part of the MMR (measles, mumps, rubella) vaccine.

- Make sure your child has the full programme of MMR immunizations.
- An attack of rubella also confers immunity, but if you plan to become pregnant, have your immunity checked first, even if you have had rubella. Make sure you are immunized, if necessary, before you conceive.

Immunity check
A simple blood test will establish your immunity to rubella.

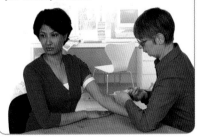

Glandular fever

Glandular fever, also known as infectious mononucleosis, is a viral illness that most commonly affects teenagers and young adults. Mainly spread by kissing, sneezing, coughing, and by sharing cups and glasses, it takes 4–8 weeks to incubate. The symptoms are a sore throat, fever, and loss of appetite and energy that persist for more than a week or two. You may also have swollen glands in your neck and sometimes in your groin and under your arms, and a headache. Glandular fever is not usually serious, and there is no specific medical treatment for it. Recovery can take 4–6 weeks, but you may feel tired for several months.

 ### See your doctor first

Arrange to see your doctor to confirm the diagnosis and check for complications.

What you can do yourself

Take plenty of rest while your immune system is fighting the virus, and use these simple measures to make yourself more comfortable.

- If you are feeling tired, rest. You may need to stay in bed for the first few days of the illness.

- Take a painkiller (see DRUG REMEDIES, right) to reduce fever and discomfort. If you have a high temperature, wear lightweight clothes and put a fan in your room.

- Drink plenty of water and fruit juices to avoid becoming dehydrated. Warm drinks will help to soothe a painful throat.

- Try gargling with warm salt water or use an analgesic gargle or spray (see DRUG REMEDIES, right) to provide temporary relief.

- Eating healthy foods may help to support your immune system (see NATURAL REMEDIES, right).

- Take steps to reduce stress while you are ill and during your recovery (see pp.20–21).

- Glandular fever can affect your liver, so don't drink alcohol until you have fully recovered.

- Don't take part in contact sports or other strenuous activities while you are ill and for at least 6–8 weeks after recovery.

- Stay away from school or work until your fever has gone and your strength and appetite are back to normal.

DRUG REMEDIES

Painkillers relieve fever and pain. Take paracetamol (see p.187) or ibuprofen (see p.184).

Gargles and throat sprays (see MOUTH AND THROAT TREATMENTS, p.186) relieve a sore throat temporarily. Dissolve half a teaspoon of salt in a glass of warm water to make a soothing gargle. Painkilling gargles and sprays reduce pain and inflammation; some numb the throat. These may not be suitable for children under 12 years.

NATURAL REMEDIES

Healthy diet Eaten as part of a balanced diet, certain nutrients are believed to help support the immune system. Boost your diet with lean meat; oily fish such as salmon, sardines, and pilchards; fresh fruit; leafy and dark green vegetables; wheatgerm; walnuts; sunflower seeds; and linseed.

Benefits of fruit
Fresh fruit is a good source of many of the vitamins that are needed to fight infection.

 ### Seek further medical advice

Arrange to see your doctor urgently if you begin to develop:

- Difficulty breathing or swallowing
- Severe headache and a stiff neck
- Chest or abdominal pain

Measles

Measles is a highly contagious viral infection that was common in children before immunization. The incubation period is about 10 days. At first your child has a hacking cough, runny nose, red eyes, and fever. After about 2–4 days, flat red or brown blotches appear on the face, and spread to cover the body and limbs. There may be small white spots inside the cheeks. Most children make a good recovery, but measles can lead to ear infections and to complications such as pneumonia and, rarely, inflammation of the brain.

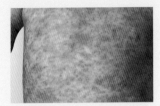

Child with measles rash

⊕ See your doctor first

Make an appointment for your child to see your doctor to confirm the diagnosis and get appropriate medical treatment.

What you can do yourself

Measles is an unpleasant illness and at first your child may feel very unwell. Try the following to reduce discomfort and distress.

● If your child has a fever, give a painkiller to reduce it (*see* DRUG REMEDIES, right). Dress your child in light clothes and put a fan in the room. Offer your child plenty of fluids throughout the day to replace water lost through sweating.

● Make sure your child rests while he or she has a raised temperature.

● Warm drinks will help to soothe a cough.

● Reduce the lighting in the room if your child's eyes are sensitive to light.

● Warm, moist air helps to soothe air passages and loosen mucus. Create a humid atmosphere by using a vaporizer, putting a damp towel on a radiator, or sitting with your child in a steamy bathroom.

● Your child will be infectious from the first signs of infection until 4 days after the rash appears, and can go back to school after that time if he or she is well and there are no complications from measles.

DRUG REMEDIES

Painkillers Paracetamol (*see* p.187) or ibuprofen (*see* p.184), which are available in various forms, will help to bring down a fever and reduce general discomfort. Your pharmacist will advise which is most suitable for your child.

PREVENTION

Immunization to protect against measles is given as part of the MMR (measles, mumps, rubella) vaccine. Make sure your child is immunized.

MMR immunization
The vaccine is given as an injection, usually into the arm.

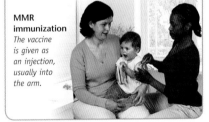

⊕ Seek further medical advice

Arrange to see your doctor urgently if your child develops:

● A severe cough and/or breathing problems
● Earache or an eye infection
● Vomiting
● Severe headaches, excessive drowsiness, and/or seizures

Influenza

Flu is a highly contagious viral illness that tends to occur in epidemics during the winter. It is spread by the coughs and sneezes of infected people and also by direct contact with contaminated articles such as handkerchiefs. About 24–48 hours after exposure to the infection, you develop a sudden fever, shivering, headache, dry cough, muscle aches, exhaustion, and sore eyes and throat. Although you will begin to feel better after 4–5 days, you may feel tired and continue coughing for several weeks.

 ## See your doctor first

Arrange to see your doctor if:

- You are frail or elderly, have heart or lung problems, have another long-term illness such as diabetes, or have recently been abroad

What you can do yourself

Although you can't shorten a bout of flu, these measures will help to relieve the worst symptoms.

- Rest for a few days and avoid any unnecessary activity. As you begin to feel better, gradually increase what you do.

- Drink plenty of fluids, such as water or fruit juice. If you don't feel like eating, have nourishing fluids such as chicken soup and broths.

 - Take a painkiller or flu remedy to relieve aches and pains (see DRUG REMEDIES, right).

- To relieve the "stuffed-up" feeling, use a steam inhalation (see PRACTICAL TECHNIQUE, p.79).

 - Warm or chilled drinks soothe a sore throat. Try making a warm honey and lemon drink (see NATURAL REMEDIES, right).

- Don't smoke or allow anyone to smoke near you.

Seek further medical advice

Arrange to see your doctor if:

- Your symptoms have not begun to clear up within a week
- You develop other symptoms, such as breathing problems, or cough up green, yellow, or bloody mucus

 ### DRUG REMEDIES

Painkillers will reduce fever and help to relieve headache and muscle aches. Take paracetamol (see p.187) or ibuprofen (see p.184).

Cold and flu remedies (see p.179) contain drugs for various symptoms. They usually include a painkiller, such as paracetamol, and a decongestant, to help you breathe more easily. Some also contain caffeine. Check the ingredients carefully. You should not use the remedies with other drugs such as painkillers because of the risk of overdose.

NATURAL REMEDIES

Honey and lemon is a soothing drink for a sore throat. Use freshly squeezed lemon juice, liquid honey, and hot water.

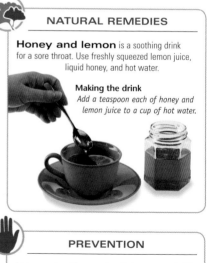

Making the drink
Add a teaspoon each of honey and lemon juice to a cup of hot water.

PREVENTION

Immunization against flu is recommended for older people and those with low immunity and/or long-term health problems. A flu jab is usually given annually in the autumn. Ask your doctor for advice.

Whooping cough

Whooping cough (pertussis) is a severe bacterial infection that was common in children before immunization. Your child may be feverish and have cold symptoms 7–10 days after contact. Then spasms of coughing develop with a typical high-pitched "whoop" as the child breathes in. Coughing is usually worse at night and may trigger vomiting. The illness can be serious in small babies.

 See also Coughing, p.102; Croup, p.138.

WARNING

Seek immediate medical help if:
- Your child becomes drowsy, has seizures, or is choking
- Your child has breathing problems, or his or her lips or tongue turn blue during a coughing spasm

 ## See your doctor first

Arrange to see your doctor immediately if you suspect your child has whooping cough.

What you can do yourself

Whooping cough can be distressing, so follow these steps to make your child more comfortable.

- Be calm and reassuring. If your child is having trouble sleeping, try to share the care at night.

- Offer plenty of clear fluids. Try honey and lemon (*see* NATURAL REMEDIES, opposite page), but don't give honey to babies under 1 year.

 - Give your child a painkiller (*see* DRUG REMEDIES, right) to reduce fever and discomfort. Don't use cough medicines – they will not help.

 - Humidifying the room (*see* PRACTICAL TECHNIQUE, right) may help to ease the cough.

- Offering your child soft, easy-to-swallow food in small portions will help to prevent vomiting.

- Keep your home free of irritants such as tobacco smoke and aerosol sprays.

 ## Seek further medical advice

Arrange to see your doctor:

- If your child's condition deteriorates
- To check that your child is fit to return to school; he or she may have coughing fits for several months after the illness

DRUG REMEDIES

Painkillers will help to reduce discomfort and bring down a fever. Give paracetamol (*see* p.187) or ibuprofen (*see* p.184), which are available in various forms. Your pharmacist will be able to advise you about which type is most suitable for your child.

Liquid paracetamol
You can give medicines containing liquid paracetamol to a child over 3 months old.

PRACTICAL TECHNIQUE

Humidifying air in a room will soothe your child's air passages and help to loosen mucus. Use one of the following methods.

- Place a humidifier by the child's bed, or hang a wet towel close to a radiator.
- Sit with your child in the bathroom and run hot water in the bath or shower to create steam.

 ## PREVENTION

An effective vaccine that protects against whooping cough is included in the childhood immunization programme. Make sure your child is immunized according to the recommended schedule.

Chickenpox

Chickenpox is a highly infectious viral illness, most common in children, that causes an intensely itchy rash of blisters. Your child may generally feel unwell, with a headache and mild fever, just before the rash develops and for the first few days afterwards. The first symptoms appear 10–21 days after contact with the infection, and most children are completely recovered 7–10 days later.

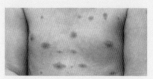
Chickenpox rash on a child

 ### See your doctor first

Arrange to see your doctor to confirm that your child has chickenpox.

What you can do yourself

Use these home treatments to make your child more comfortable and help prevent scratching, which can cause scars.

- If your child has a fever, take steps to reduce it (see FEVER IN CHILDREN, p.135). Offer your child plenty to drink throughout the day.

- Soothe itching by giving your child lukewarm baths twice a day. Try adding sodium bicarbonate (baking soda) or an oatmeal lotion to the bath water (see NATURAL REMEDIES, right).

- An antihistamine will reduce itching and help your child to sleep at night. You can also soothe the skin with a crotamiton cream or lotion, or calamine lotion (see DRUG REMEDIES, right).

- Cut your child's nails short to reduce damage from scratching. Give him or her cotton gloves to wear at night to prevent scratching during sleep.

- To soothe spots in your child's mouth, get him or her to rinse with half a teaspoon of salt in a cup of warm water, taking care that he or she does not swallow the solution. Encourage your child to keep brushing his or her teeth as normal.

- Your child will be more comfortable in light, loose, non-itchy clothing. Avoid wool.

- Keep your child away from school, and away from any woman who may be pregnant, for 5 days from the time when the blisters first appear.

NATURAL REMEDIES

Sodium bicarbonate (see p.188) reduces itching. Add 2 tablespoons to a bath one-third full.

Oatmeal products (see p.186) moisturize the skin; lotions can be used instead of soap.

DRUG REMEDIES

Antihistamines (see p.178) will help to relieve itching. Try a liquid sedative brand if itching makes sleep difficult for your child.

Crotamiton preparations (see p.180) are creams or lotions applied 2–3 times a day. Keep them away from eyes or broken skin. Don't use them on children under 3 without consulting your doctor.

Calamine lotion (see p.179) is cooling and helps to dry up blisters. Use it as needed.

Applying calamine
Use cotton wool and count the spots with your child as you dab on the lotion.

 ### Seek further medical advice

Arrange to see your doctor again if your child develops:

- Pus-filled spots and/or blisters near the eyes
- Earache or headache, breathing problems, drowsiness, or convulsions

Shingles

Shingles is caused by reactivation of the chickenpox virus, which lies dormant in anyone who has had chickenpox. It begins with pain or tingling in an area of skin on one side of your body or face, followed by a rash of small, fluid-filled blisters. You may also have a headache and fever. The blisters scab over and heal within a few weeks, but the area may be painful for months afterwards. Shingles is more common in later life. Stress, ill health, or sunlight can trigger an attack, but you can't catch shingles from contact with chickenpox.

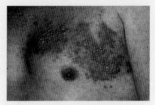

Shingles rash

See your doctor first

Arrange to see your doctor to confirm that you have shingles. See your doctor urgently if shingles has developed close to an eye.

What you can do yourself

Use these home treatments to make yourself feel better while you get over an attack of shingles.

- Rest as much as you can to speed your recovery.
- While you have a fever, drink plenty of fluids.

- Take a painkiller to relieve pain, headache, and fever (*see* DRUG REMEDIES, right). A cold compress (a cloth soaked in ice-cold water) may help relieve pain and tingling in your skin.

- If you have blisters on your body, take lukewarm baths 2–3 times a day. Add sodium bicarbonate (baking soda) or use an oatmeal product (*see* NATURAL REMEDIES, right) to soothe your skin. Wash any blisters on your face gently with soap and water.
- Until all the blisters have dried up, avoid contact with anyone who has not had chickenpox, because they could catch the virus from you.

Seek further medical advice

Arrange to see your doctor again if:

- Your blisters become pus-filled and spread
- You develop severe headaches or vomiting
- Painkillers do not control the pain, or pain persists after the blisters have cleared

DRUG REMEDIES

Painkillers will relieve fever as well as pain. Use paracetamol (*see* p.187), aspirin (*see* p.179), or ibuprofen (*see* p.184). If you need stronger pain relief, take paracetamol and codeine (*see* p.187). Ask your pharmacist for advice.

NATURAL REMEDIES

Sodium bicarbonate (*see* p.188) can also help to reduce itching. Add 4 tablespoons (about one cup) to a bath two-thirds full.

Oatmeal products (*see* p.186) are soothing for itchy, blistered skin. Either add oatmeal oil to your bath or use the lotion instead of soap.

PREVENTION

Preventing attacks If you are susceptible to shingles, try the following measures:

- If shingles tends to develop when you are under stress, try using deep breathing exercises and muscle relaxation techniques to help you relax (*see* PRACTICAL TECHNIQUES, pp.20–21).
- Be careful to protect your skin from strong sunlight (*see* PREVENTION: SAFETY IN THE SUN, p.47).

SKIN, HAIR, AND NAIL PROBLEMS

Impetigo

Impetigo is a common skin infection that mainly affects children. It can appear anywhere on the body but most often develops on the face, especially around the nose and mouth. Red, weepy sores develop; the sores then blister and burst, and dry out to form an itchy, honey-coloured crust. Caused by bacterial infection, impetigo is highly contagious and is spread by touch. The bacteria are present in small numbers on healthy skin, but impetigo tends to develop when there are minor cuts or grazes that allow the bacteria to get under the skin.

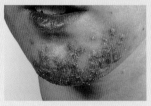

Impetigo sores

 ### See your doctor first

Make an appointment to see your doctor to confirm impetigo. The doctor will probably prescribe antibiotics.

What you can do yourself

Impetigo usually clears up promptly with antibiotic treatment, but the following measures will speed recovery and reduce the risk of the sores spreading.

 ● Wash the affected area carefully (*see* PRACTICAL TECHNIQUE, right).

● Make sure your child has towels and face cloths for his or her own use. Change them daily and wash them in very hot water. Encourage your child to wash his or her hands frequently, drying them properly each time.

● Remind your child not to touch or pick the scabs or suck his or her fingers. Trim his or her nails to help prevent scratching.

● If your doctor prescribes an antibiotic drug or cream, make sure you give your child the complete course. Do not stop as soon as the impetigo appears to be better.

● Keep your child away from other children until there is no longer any crusting over the sores. Your child can then return to school or nursery.

 ### PRACTICAL TECHNIQUE

Washing infected areas Use the following procedure to soften and remove crusts and help the skin to heal. (If you are using an antibiotic ointment, do this before you apply the ointment.)

● Soak the affected area by applying a clean face cloth soaked in warm water. Hold it over the skin for 1–2 minutes, being careful not to rub the rash. Pat the skin dry with a towel. Repeat this several times a day, washing your hands afterwards.
● Do not cover the blisters. They will heal better if you leave them exposed to the air.

 ### Seek further medical advice

Arrange to see your doctor again if:

● The sores spread or enlarge
● The impetigo rash has not begun to clear within a few days
● Your child develops a fever or starts to pass red- or brown-coloured urine

Scabies

Scabies is an infestation caused by a mite that burrows just under the skin surface. At first you will have intense itching, which is worse at night. You may then notice little bumps and tiny, pencil-like lines (burrows); these usually develop between the fingers and toes and on the elbows and wrists, but may occur anywhere on your skin. Scabies is troublesome rather than serious. Anyone can catch it, regardless of age and personal hygiene, through any type of skin-to-skin contact or simply by sharing bedding, towels, or clothing.

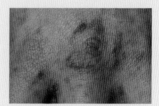

Scabies infestation on a hand and fingers

See your doctor first

Make an appointment to see your doctor if:

- You are not sure that you have scabies
- You are pregnant or breastfeeding
- A baby under 6 months has scabies

What you can do yourself

For best results, start scabies treatment as soon as the symptoms appear. This may be anything up to 6 weeks after infestation, and the itching can last for several weeks.

- Use a cream or lotion for treating scabies (see DRUG REMEDIES, right).

- You can relieve itching with a skin cream or lotion and/or take an antihistamine if itching is making it difficult for you to sleep (see DRUG REMEDIES, right).

- Make sure other people in the home and close friends are treated, even if they are not showing signs of scabies, because they can have the infestation without symptoms.

- Scabies mites can live for 1–2 days in clothes and bedding. To kill the mites, wash clothes, bed linen, and towels in hot water and dry in a tumble dryer if possible. Wash personal items such as hairbrushes as well. Items that cannot be washed easily can be placed in a sealed plastic bag for at least 72 hours, which will kill the mites.

DRUG REMEDIES

Scabies lotions (see p.188) usually contain the insecticide substances malathion or permethrin. Ask your pharmacist to suggest a suitable preparation. Apply the treatment to your entire body, including your scalp, face, ears, and neck. Trim your nails short and apply it underneath your nail tips. Permethrin preparations should be left on for 8–12 hours and malathion preparations for 24 hours before washing off. A second application a week later is recommended.

Antihistamines (see p.178) can help to relieve itching. Sedative types make you drowsy, so are particularly useful at night.

Creams Crotamiton cream (see p.180) or calamine lotion (see p.179) help to relieve itching.

Relieving itching
Itching can persist for several weeks after the infestation has cleared, so you may need to continue using anti-itching cream.

Seek further medical advice

Arrange to see your doctor if:

- You are still itching more than 2 weeks after finishing your course of treatment
- The rash becomes sore and starts to ooze

Hives

Hives, or urticaria, is an intensely itchy rash of white or yellow swellings (weals) surrounded by red, inflamed skin. It is usually caused by an allergic reaction, which can be triggered by a range of factors, such as certain foods or medicines, insect bites, or stings. People with hay fever or asthma are more susceptible. Hives can also be caused by stress, or have no obvious cause.

 See also Anaphylactic shock, p.159.

> ### WARNING
> Seek immediate medical help if you have hives and:
> • You become breathless, wheezy, or hoarse
> • Your lips or tongue swell and/or you have difficulty swallowing

See your doctor first

Make an appointment to see your doctor to confirm that you have hives and/or to check whether you are taking medication that could be triggering the attack.

What you can do yourself

Hives is extremely uncomfortable, but the following simple measures will help to relieve irritation and soothe the skin. Attacks are usually short-lived, but some people have persistent symptoms.

 • Take an antihistamine to reduce itching and swelling (*see* DRUG REMEDIES, right).

• Have a cool shower to reduce the redness and "heat" of the rash. Alternatively, hold a cool compress (a clean face cloth soaked in cool water and wrung out) against the rash for a few minutes at a time. Keep reapplying for about 30 minutes.

 • You can also relieve itching with calamine lotion, or with a cream or lotion containing crotamiton (*see* DRUG REMEDIES, right).

 • Try an oatmeal bath oil (*see* NATURAL REMEDIES, right) to relieve itchy skin.

• Minimize irritation by wearing loose-fitting, lightweight clothes made of natural fibres.

Seek further medical advice

Arrange to see your doctor again if:

• Hives is not responding to treatment

DRUG REMEDIES

Antihistamines (*see* p.178) control allergic swelling and itching. You may need to try several types to find out which works best for you. The drug may need to be taken regularly for a prolonged attack of hives. Ask your pharmacist for advice.

Calamine lotion (*see* p.179) is a soothing preparation with a cooling effect. Using a pad of cotton wool, dab it on to the rash 2–3 times a day.

Crotamiton preparations (*see* p.180) are creams or lotions that can relieve itching for 6–10 hours. Apply them 2–3 times a day, but not around the eyes or on broken skin. Don't use them on children under 3 without consulting your doctor.

NATURAL REMEDIES

Oatmeal products (*see* p.186) are often effective for soothing itchy skin. Add oatmeal oil to lukewarm bath water and soak for 10–20 minutes.

PREVENTION

Preventing hives If you have recurrent attacks, try these measures to prevent them.

• Keep a diary of attacks, and try to identify any foods, medicines, or other factors that may trigger them. Once you find a trigger, you can try to avoid it.
• If you think stress is a contributory factor, try self-help techniques (*see* STRESS, pp.20–21).

Acne

Many teenagers have acne, and for some it is a distressing and persistent problem. Outbreaks of pimples, blackheads, whiteheads, and cysts occur on the face and sometimes on the chest and back. The cause is a surge of hormones during puberty that stimulates the oil-producing glands in the skin, making them prone to blockage and infection. Acne tends to clear up over time, but the spots may leave scars. Attacks of acne in adult life can be triggered by factors such as stress, changes in the weather, and using certain cosmetics.

What you can do yourself

There are various ways to tackle acne. Start treatment early to reduce the risk of scarring.

- Try a treatment containing benzoyl peroxide to reduce pimples (*see* DRUG REMEDIES, right).

- Gently wash affected areas twice a day with lukewarm water and a non-oily, perfume-free soap. Shampoo your hair daily and keep your hair off your face. Don't use products such as conditioners.

- Avoid covering affected areas with tight-fitting clothing, and do not wear hats.

- Don't squeeze spots – they may get infected and spread. Take care not to nick spots when shaving.

- Avoid oil-based cosmetics and creams and opt for non-comedogenic products, which do not block pores. Go without make-up for 1 or 2 days a week.

- Try not to rub or touch your face absent-mindedly while you are absorbed in something such as watching TV or reading a book. Keep the phone away from your face when talking.

- Include plenty of healthy foods such as fruit and vegetables in your diet (*see* NATURAL REMEDIES, right).

- If stress makes your acne worse, try strategies that help reduce stress in your life (*see* pp.20–21).

Seek medical advice

Arrange to see your doctor if:

- Your acne has not improved, or is spreading and is red and weepy, after you have used self-help remedies for 2 months
- You are a woman, and you are also growing facial hair and having irregular periods

DRUG REMEDIES

Benzoyl peroxide (*see* p.179), used every day, is an effective treatment for mild to moderate acne. It reduces inflammation, helps destroy bacteria, and prevents new spots from forming. However, it may take up to 2 months before your skin responds to treatment. Use gel or lotion if you have oily skin; use cream for dry skin. Start with a low-strength type and go on to a higher strength if necessary. Continue the treatment until your acne clears up. Don't use benzoyl peroxide near your mouth or eyes.

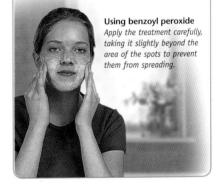

Using benzoyl peroxide
Apply the treatment carefully, taking it slightly beyond the area of the spots to prevent them from spreading.

NATURAL REMEDIES

Healthy foods are believed to support the immune system and maintain healthy skin. Boost your diet with lean meat, oily fish such as salmon, fruit, leafy and dark green vegetables, wheatgerm, walnuts, sunflower seeds, and linseed.

Eczema

Eczema causes patches of dry, intensely itchy skin, which usually appear on the face, hands, wrists, and scalp, and in the creases of the knees and elbows. Repeated scratching may leave the skin cracked and open to infection. Eczema is often linked to allergies and asthma. It usually develops in infancy and disappears by the early teenage years, but adults may have relapses triggered by factors such as stress, house dust mites, and some foods.

 See also Stress, pp.20–21; Hay fever, p.80; Food intolerance, p.113.

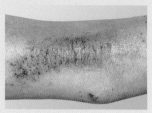
Eczema on the inside of an arm

See your doctor first

Make an appointment to see your doctor even if you are fairly sure that you have eczema.

What you can do yourself

Although there is no cure for eczema, you can take these steps to help control the symptoms.

 • Bathe only once a day using warm not hot water, and don't use perfumed bath products. Use a moisturizer instead of soap or add an emollient bath additive to the bath. Afterwards, apply moisturizer to soften and seal moisture into your skin. Reapply it generously throughout the day to the affected areas (*see* DRUG REMEDIES, right).

• Trim your nails or put on cotton gloves at night to prevent scratching. Try taking a sedative antihistamine to relieve itching and help you sleep (*see* DRUG REMEDIES, right).

• Wear cotton clothing next to your skin and avoid synthetic fabrics and wool. Wash clothes in non-biological soap powders, and rinse them well.

 • For small, resistant patches of eczema, use a mild hydrocortisone cream to relieve inflammation (*see* DRUG REMEDIES, right).

Seek further medical advice

Arrange to see your doctor again if:

• The eczema is not improving with treatment after a week, or is red, weepy, hot, or painful

DRUG REMEDIES

Moisturizers (*see* p.186) can be used instead of soap for washing. Rub aqueous cream or emulsifying ointment on your skin, rinse well, and pat yourself dry. Apply aqueous cream liberally to patches of eczema throughout the day.

Emollient bath additives (*see* p.181) contain a light liquid paraffin that soothes and cleans the skin. Soak in the bath for 10–20 minutes and pat yourself dry gently to keep the emollient on your skin.

Antihistamines (*see* p.178), in liquid form for children and as tablets for adults, relieve itching; the sedative brands will also help you sleep.

Hydrocortisone cream (*see* p.184) can be used for eczema but for no longer than a week. Apply sparingly, but not to your face unless your doctor tells you otherwise. Do not use the cream on children under 10 without medical advice.

PREVENTION

Avoiding triggers Certain factors can trigger eczema. Try to avoid any that affect you.

• Wear cotton-lined rubber or disposable gloves when using chemicals such as detergents and dyes.
• Follow practical advice on reducing allergens in your home (*see* PREVENTION, p.103).
• If you suspect that certain foods trigger eczema, try excluding them temporarily (*see* PRACTICAL TECHNIQUE: ELIMINATION DIET, p.113). Consult a doctor or dietitian before eliminating foods from a child's diet.

Psoriasis

In psoriasis, patches of red, thickened skin with silvery scales develop, usually on your elbows, knees, scalp, and trunk. These areas can be itchy and painful. Your nails may become rough and pitted, and, less commonly, a form of arthritis develops. Psoriasis can be a persistent problem, and tends to run in families. Stress, infections such as a sore throat, and skin injuries may trigger an attack or make it worse.

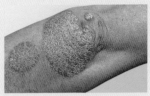

Psoriasis on an elbow

 See also Disfigured or brittle nails, p.53.

 ## See your doctor first

Make an appointment to see your doctor if you think that you have psoriasis.

What you can do yourself

The following measures may be all you need to treat a mild case of psoriasis. Check with your doctor before using them with prescribed treatment.

 • Take a daily bath in warm water to soak off the scales. Try using a coal tar preparation (*see* DRUG REMEDIES, right) to soften the scales.

 • Apply a moisturizer to lubricate and soften scaly patches of skin (*see* DRUG REMEDIES, right).

 • Don't scratch or rub patches of thickened skin. Using an oatmeal bath oil, or applying an aloe vera cream or gel, may help to reduce itchiness (*see* NATURAL REMEDIES, right).

• Sunshine can help to improve psoriasis but be careful not to burn. Sunburn can make it worse.

• If stress is making your psoriasis worse, try some deep breathing and muscle relaxation exercises (*see* PRACTICAL TECHNIQUES, pp.20–21).

 ## Seek further medical advice

Arrange to see your doctor again if:

• Your psoriasis is not controlled by treatment
• Large areas of skin become red and inflamed, and you have a fever and feel unwell
• You develop joint pains

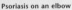 ### DRUG REMEDIES

Coal tar preparations (*see* p.179) help to control psoriasis but have a strong smell. Add a coal tar solution to a daily bath; apply a cream (usually 1–3 times daily); and use a coal tar shampoo. If you have thick scales on your scalp, use coal tar combined with salicylic acid to soften and remove them. If your skin becomes irritated, discontinue use. Coal tar makes skin more sensitive to ultraviolet light, so avoid exposing skin to sunlight after use.

Moisturizers (*see* p.186), such as aqueous cream, should be rubbed gently into the skin as often as possible to relieve itching and loosen scales.

 ### NATURAL REMEDIES

Oatmeal bath oils (*see* p.186) help to soften scaly plaques and relieve itching.

Aloe vera creams and gels (*see* p.177) may help to reduce dryness and itching in psoriasis. There is some evidence for their effectiveness but ask your doctor for advice before using them.

Using aloe vera
Apply aloe vera gel or cream thinly to irritated and itchy patches of skin and rub in lightly.

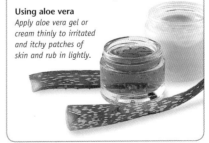

Rosacea

Rosacea is a flush or rash on your chin, nose, cheeks, and forehead. You may also have small bumps and pimples on your cheeks, sore eyes and eyelids, and, more rarely, a swollen, red nose. Rosacea is triggered by factors such as emotional stress, alcohol, or hot, spicy food. Flare-ups are due to inflammation of the tiny blood vessels under the skin but why rosacea develops in the first place is unknown. The condition seems to run in families, is more common in women aged 30–55, and may be lifelong.

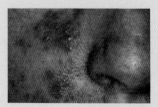
Rosacea rash on cheek

 See your doctor first

Make an appointment to see your doctor if you think you have rosacea.

What you can do yourself

Flare-ups are usually caused by something that makes you flush or overheat. There are several things you can do to reduce the symptoms.

- Put a cold compress (a face cloth soaked in ice-cold water) on the flushed areas to cool your skin.

- Some foods and drinks trigger attacks. Try to identify which, if any, are affecting you (*see* PRACTICAL TECHNIQUE, right).

- Use mild cleansers and avoid any that contain alcohol. Don't rub your face hard or use a face cloth.

- Bathe or shower in tepid, rather than hot, water.

- Wear cotton rather than wool and dress in layers so you can remove a layer if you begin to feel hot.

- To minimize redness, try a green-tinted foundation; choose one that is specially formulated for sensitive skin. Camouflage creams are also available but you may need specialist advice on selecting and applying them.

- Use a moisturizer to protect your skin against the drying effects of cold weather.

- If you are a man with rosacea, use an electric shaver rather than wet shave.

PRACTICAL TECHNIQUE

Identifying trigger substances
This should help you to avoid particular foods and drinks, such as coffee, alcohol, and spicy food, that can cause flare-ups of rosacea.

- Keep a diary of your symptoms and what you have eaten when they occur.
- Try eliminating any suspect foods or drinks for up to 6 weeks to see if there is an improvement.
- Reintroduce foods and drinks one at a time, noting which provoke an attack and need to be avoided.

PREVENTION

Avoiding attacks If you are prone to flushes, following the advice given here may help to reduce the frequency and severity of attacks.

- Sunlight can cause flare-ups, so stay in the shade on hot summer days and wear a hat. When you are in the sun, use a sunscreen; a titanium dioxide sunblock (*see* DRUG REMEDIES: SUNSCREENS AND SUNBLOCKS, p.47) is less likely to irritate your skin.
- Avoid rapid changes of temperature – for example, going straight from the cold outdoors into a hot room.
- If you tend to have flare-ups of rosacea when you are feeling under stress, try practising deep breathing exercises and muscle relaxation techniques (*see* PRACTICAL TECHNIQUES, pp.20–21).

Dry skin

When your skin lacks moisture it tends to be itchy and flaky. It may look red, rough, and scaly and, in severe cases, become cracked and inflamed. You are most likely to develop dry skin on your lower legs, arms, and the backs of your hands because these areas produce less of the natural oils that seal moisture into the skin. Your skin also becomes drier as you get older and during the menopause. You may develop sore, rough, chapped skin on your face in dry, cold weather, or if your face gets wet repeatedly and is not dried properly.

What you can do yourself

There are plenty of easy-to-use remedies that reduce the discomfort of dry, itchy skin and improve its appearance. Use the following measures.

● Have baths rather than showers (which tend to strip oils from the skin) no more than once a day in warm, rather than hot, water. Don't use perfumed or medicated bath products or soaps.

● Use moisturizing cream or ointment instead of soap or add an emollient bath additive to your bath (see DRUG REMEDIES, right).

● After your bath, apply a moisturizing cream (see DRUG REMEDIES, right). Reapply it frequently to exposed areas such as your hands and face, especially after washing or if you are outdoors for long periods in cold weather. Keep tubes of cream around the house and at work to use during the day.

● Alternatively, use a bath oil containing oatmeal (see NATURAL REMEDIES, right).

PREVENTION

Preventing dryness If your skin tends to get dry or chapped, try the following measures.

● Don't overheat your home. In centrally heated rooms keep the air moist by fitting humidifying devices to radiators, or put bowls of water near them.
● Wear rubber gloves for household cleaning and gloves for gardening and other outdoor activities.
● Limit sunbathing. Use a sunscreen (see DRUG REMEDIES: SUNSCREENS AND SUNBLOCKS, p.47) when you are out in the sun. At high altitudes, use a sunscreen formulated for skiing or a total sunblock.
● Rinse your laundry well and don't use fabric conditioners; they may irritate your skin.

DRUG REMEDIES

Emollient bath additives (see p.181) contain substances such as light liquid paraffin that disperse in water to make a soothing, milky bath that also cleans the skin. Soak for 10–20 minutes and pat yourself dry gently to keep the emollient on your skin.

Moisturizers (see p.186) can be used for washing and to protect and soothe dry skin. Use aqueous cream or emulsifying ointment in the bath and when you wash. Rinse off thoroughly, pat your skin dry, and then apply more aqueous cream.

Aqueous cream
Apply aqueous cream liberally to your skin while it is still moist after a bath.

NATURAL REMEDIES

Oatmeal bath oil (see OATMEAL PRODUCTS, p.186) is soothing and moisturizing for dry, itchy skin. Add it to a warm bath and soak for 10–20 minutes.

Seek medical advice

Arrange to see your doctor if:

● You still have dry, chapped skin after trying the measures described above
● Your skin becomes inflamed and bleeds

Corns and calluses

Prolonged pressure or friction on the feet or hands can cause patches of hard skin – corns or calluses – to form. Corns tend to develop over the toe joints or between toes, often as a result of badly fitting shoes. Calluses may occur on the soles of your feet, usually due to uneven pressure when walking, or on your hands if you do heavy manual work or play a musical instrument. Corns and calluses protect the soft skin beneath, so you may not need to remove them unless they are painful.

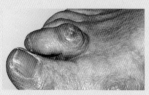

Corn on toe joint

See your doctor or chiropodist first

Make an appointment to see your doctor or a chiropodist if you have corns and calluses and you also have diabetes or suffer from poor circulation.

What you can do yourself

First find out what has caused the corn or callus, because it will be easier to treat once the source of friction has been removed. Take the following steps to relieve the problem.

- Use a foam wedge to relieve pressure on corns between the toes, and corn pads (small rings of sponge) to protect corns in other areas. Hydrocolloid corn plasters will help to cushion and soften the skin (*see* DRUG REMEDIES, right).

- Soak the corn or callus in warm, soapy water for 10 minutes each day, then use a pumice stone to gently rub away the hard skin.

- Never cut or shave corns yourself. Instead, you can apply salicylic acid to soften the thickened skin gradually (*see* DRUG REMEDIES, right).

Seek further medical advice

Arrange to see your doctor if:

- Your corn or callus does not disappear with self-help measures
- The skin is becoming painful, red, swollen, or weepy, or an ulcer develops

DRUG REMEDIES

Hydrocolloid plasters (*see* p.183) for corns and calluses contain a substance that absorbs moisture released by the skin. This forms a gel that cushions the area and also softens the skin so that the corn or callus can be removed easily.

Salicylic acid gels, lotions, or ointments (*see* p.187) can be used to soften calluses and corns, making them easier to remove. Products containing salicylic acid may burn surrounding skin, so apply them with care and follow the instructions carefully. Alternatively, use corn pads or plasters, which apply salicylic acid directly to the corn.

Moisturizers (*see* p.186) soften the skin, so calluses are less likely to develop. Apply aqueous cream or emulsifying ointment to the hands and feet after washing and during the day.

PREVENTION

Preventing corns and calluses

The following measures will help to protect your hands and feet from friction and pressure.

- Wear comfortable shoes that fit properly. Avoid high heels and pointed shoes. Make sure worn-down soles and heels are repaired promptly.

- If your soles are prone to calluses, cushion them with hydrocolloid plasters (*see* DRUG REMEDIES, above) or padding inside your shoe.
- Use a moisturizer regularly to keep your skin soft (*see* DRUG REMEDIES, above).
- Wear padded gloves when using tools or machinery.
- If you play a stringed instrument, it may help to put plasters on your fingertips for protection.

Warts and verrucas

Warts are small, round growths on the skin that have a rough, cauliflower-like appearance and, sometimes, tiny black spots in the centre. They are caused by a virus, are contagious, and tend to be most common in children and young adults. Warts are most likely to develop on your hands or on the soles of your feet; those that occur on the feet are called verrucas. They do not usually hurt, but verrucas may be painful because walking puts pressure on them – it may feel rather like having a pebble in your shoe.

 ## See your doctor first

Make an appointment to see your doctor if:

● You are not entirely certain that a new growth on your skin is a wart
● You have warts on your face or around the anus or genitals: these need special treatment

What you can do yourself

Most warts disappear eventually, but it can take a long time – sometimes years. Prompt treatment may, however, help to prevent them from spreading or hurting and can clear them up completely.

 ● A wart remover is usually effective (*see* DRUG REMEDIES, right).

● Follow a treatment regime using a pumice stone and salicylic acid wart remover until your wart has disappeared (*see* PRACTICAL TECHNIQUE, right).

● A soft insole inside your shoe may help to reduce the discomfort of a verruca.

● Don't scratch or pick at your warts – this may make them spread. Nailbiting may also spread the infection, so try not to do it (*see* NAILBITING, p.54).

 ## Seek further medical advice

Arrange to see your doctor if:

● Your wart does not respond to treatment
● The wart changes in appearance, bleeds, or becomes red, hot, and painful

DRUG REMEDIES

Wart and verucca treatments
(*see* p.189) contain either salicylic acid, which softens warts so that they can be removed easily, or chemicals that freeze warts, causing them to fall off in about 10–14 days. Make sure that you apply these products only to the wart and not the surrounding skin.

PRACTICAL TECHNIQUE

Treating a wart You can remove a wart gradually by soaking it, rubbing it with a pumice stone, and applying a salicylic acid wart remover. Instructions for use vary, but many are used as follows.

1 *First soak the wart for a few minutes in warm water to soften it. Then use a pumice stone to rub the surface of the wart gently. This will help to remove dead skin.*

Rub away dead skin from the surface of the wart

2 *Isolate the wart with a corn pad, or shield the surrounding skin with petroleum jelly. Apply the wart remover, then cover the treated wart with a plaster.*

Keep wart remover away from surrounding skin

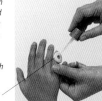

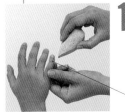

3 *Once a week, rub away the treated surface with the pumice stone. Treat the wart until it disappears. (This may take up to 12 weeks.)*

Athlete's foot and jock itch

These are common fungal infections. Athlete's foot affects the skin between the toes, making it cracked, sore, and itchy with peeling areas. It may spread to the soles and toenails. Jock itch is an itchy, scaly, red rash in the groin, more common in men. Both infections thrive in warm, sweaty conditions. You can catch them from contact with an infected person or sharing items such as towels and footwear.

 See also Ringworm, p.48; Disfigured or brittle nails, p.53.

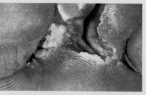

Athlete's foot between the toes

What you can do yourself

Both infections are easy to treat yourself. Keep using the good hygiene practices outlined below to help prevent fungal infections recurring.

Athlete's foot

 ● Treat the infection with an antifungal cream and/or powder (*see* DRUG REMEDIES, right).

● Wash your feet twice daily, making sure you dry thoroughly between your toes afterwards. Use a separate towel just for drying your feet, and launder the towel frequently.

● Wear socks made from natural fibres and change them at least once a day. Women should avoid wearing tights and stockings, especially those that cramp the feet.

● Wear well-ventilated shoes made from natural rather than synthetic materials; open-toed sandals are particularly good.

● Wear flip-flops when walking around communal changing areas, such as at swimming baths.

Jock itch

● Apply an antifungal treatment to the infected area (*see* DRUG REMEDIES, right).

● Wash your groin regularly, drying it thoroughly but avoiding chafing. Use a separate towel to dry this area, and launder the towel frequently.

● Don't wear tight-fitting trousers or underwear, or underwear made from synthetic fabrics. Cotton pants or boxer shorts are best. Change them daily.

DRUG REMEDIES

Antifungal drugs (*see* p.178), such as clotrimazole, miconazole, or terbinafine, are used to treat athlete's foot and jock itch. They are available as a cream or a fine powder spray (which is usually easier to apply) and should be applied as directed. The infection should start to clear up within a week, although it may take several weeks longer to disappear completely. To help treat athlete's foot, you can also dust inside your shoes and socks with an antifungal foot powder.

Powder spray
Apply the powder after washing and drying your feet carefully. Spray generously, paying particular attention to areas between the toes.

 ### Seek medical advice

Arrange to see your doctor if:

● The affected area becomes hot and red, or starts weeping
● The infection does not clear up after you have tried self-help treatment

Boils

A boil begins as a small, red, painful lump under the skin, which swells as pus builds up inside. The area is usually warm to the touch and throbs. The cause is most commonly an infection in a hair follicle or oil gland in the skin; the buttocks, thighs, armpits, face, and neck are particularly susceptible. Most boils come to a head and burst, releasing pus, after which the skin heals. Some boils, however, gradually subside without bursting. Sometimes, a cluster of connected boils forms; this is known as a carbuncle.

 See your doctor first

Make an appointment to see your doctor if:

- You think you have a carbuncle
- You have diabetes

What you can do yourself

There are several simple measures that you can take to reduce discomfort and speed up healing.

- Take a painkiller such as paracetamol if the boil is painful (*see* DRUG REMEDIES, right).
- Wash the area thoroughly every day. Dry it well.

- Help to bring the boil to a head by applying a warm compress several times a day (*see* PRACTICAL TECHNIQUE, right).

- Don't squeeze the boil or try to burst it with a needle because this may spread the infection; leave it to burst or subside by itself.

- If the boil has burst, cover the area with a gauze dressing. Wash the area thoroughly and change the dressing regularly until the skin has healed.

- Keep your own towels and face cloths separate to avoid spreading the infection to other people.

- If bedding or clothing comes into contact with the boil, wash it in very hot, preferably boiling, water.

- Wash your hands thoroughly and dry them on a clean towel before handling food. You should also make sure the boil is covered with a plaster or other dressing. The bacteria that cause boils can also cause food poisoning.

- Avoid contact sports until the boil has gone.

DRUG REMEDIES

Painkillers, such as paracetamol (*see* p.187), can relieve the pain of an inflamed or irritating boil.

PRACTICAL TECHNIQUE

Applying a warm compress
Use this treatment up to 4 times a day to help bring the boil to a head and encourage it to burst.

- Soak a clean cloth in a bowl of warm water, then wring it out and place it over the boil. Soaking the compress repeatedly to rewarm it, continue to reapply it for about 30 minutes.
- Cover the boil with a gauze dressing.
- Keep using the compress for a few days after the boil has burst, to encourage it to drain.

Applying heat
Heat a cloth in warm water and hold it over the boil until it cools.

 Seek further medical advice

Arrange to see your doctor if:

- The boil has not begun to disappear after a week of using self-help measures
- It becomes very painful and/or enlarges
- You are getting recurrent boils
- You develop a fever and feel generally unwell

Heat rash and sunburn

Heat rash, also known as prickly heat, is an itchy, red, pimply rash that may develop around your neck and on your chest, back, armpits, and groin in hot or humid weather, particularly during exercise. Babies who overheat because they are dressed too warmly, or because of a fever, are particularly susceptible to heat rash. Sunburn is the result of overexposure to sunshine or to ultraviolet rays on a sunbed. If you are mildly burnt you will have red, sore skin on areas such as your shoulders, arms, thighs, back, and nose, which may begin to itch and peel a few days later. More severe sunburn can cause blistering and pain. Although you are most likely to burn in hot summer sun, you can also burn on an overcast day, in water, or at high altitudes, for example. Babies, children, and fair-skinned people with red or blond hair and blue eyes are most at risk.

 See also Fever (children), p.135; Fever (babies), p.142.

See your doctor first

Arrange to see a doctor immediately if:

- You are not sure that a baby has heat rash, or a baby has a rash with fever
- You have severe sunburn with extensive blistering, and/or feel unwell, with vomiting, fever, confusion, or headaches
- A child or baby has sunburn

What you can do yourself

You can treat an attack of heat rash or a case of mild sunburn with the following measures. They will make your skin feel more comfortable and help to speed your recovery.

Heat rash
- Loosen or remove your clothing and find a cool place to sit, such as an air-conditioned room. If available, use a fan to help cool yourself down, and avoid any activity that might make you sweat.

- Have plenty of cool, non-alcoholic drinks.

- Apply a cold compress to affected areas. Soak a sponge or face cloth in cold water, wring it out, and apply it to your skin. Use it as often as needed.

 - If your baby develops heat rash, take immediate steps to cool him or her down (*see* PRACTICAL TECHNIQUE, right).

- To soothe dry, itchy skin, try taking frequent, lukewarm baths with oatmeal bath oil (*see* p.186). Pat your skin dry afterwards.

 PRACTICAL TECHNIQUE

Treating a baby with heat rash
A baby with heat rash needs to be cooled down promptly. The rash should then disappear.

- Take off your baby's clothes and nappy and lay him or her on a cotton sheet or towel to let the air circulate around the skin. Leave your baby to kick freely until he or she cools down.
- Don't use ointments, lotions, or powders because they may block the pores and aggravate the rash.
- If your baby has a fever, give plenty of fluids and take steps to reduce it (*see* FEVER [BABIES], p.142).

Cooling down
Once your baby is undressed, the air will help to cool his or her skin.

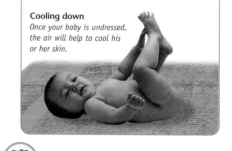

NATURAL REMEDIES

Aloe vera (*see* p.177) is found in many after-sun lotions and is also available as a gel. It has soothing properties that help to cool sunburnt skin and relieve dryness and irritation. However, don't use gels or cream to treat heat rash.

What you can do yourself *continued...*

- While you have a heat rash, don't use antiperspirants, perfumes, lotions, or creams, as they may irritate your skin or block your pores.

- When the weather is warm, wear lightweight, loose clothes made of natural fibres such as cotton.

- If you are prone to heat rash, acclimatize yourself gradually whenever you move from a cool climate to a hot one. Increase the time you spend in the heat over several days.

- To prevent heat rash in a baby, avoid overdressing or using too many blankets. (Check by feeling the back of your baby's neck – it should be warm but not sweaty.) On hot days, keep your baby in cool, shady areas and give him or her plenty to drink.

Sunburn

- Stay out of the sun while you have sunburn. If you do go outdoors, wear cool, lightweight clothes that cover the burns completely.

- Don't pick at peeling skin and leave any blisters to burst on their own.

- Have a cool bath and add about 4 tablespoons of sodium bicarbonate (*see* p.188) to the bath water. Pat yourself dry with a soft towel.

- You may find a cold compress soothing. Soak a soft cloth in cold water, wring it out, and apply it gently to your sunburnt skin. Repeat as often as you need to throughout the day.

- Calamine lotion may help to cool sunburnt skin (*see* DRUG REMEDIES, right).

- Try an aloe vera lotion or gel to soothe your skin (*see* NATURAL REMEDIES, opposite page). Wait until the skin has been cooled down before applying moisturizers, as they hold in the heat of the burn.

Seek further medical advice

Arrange to see your doctor if:

- A heat rash does not fade within 2–3 days
- A baby is still feverish after you have used cooling-down methods

DRUG REMEDIES

Calamine lotion (*see* p.179) has a cooling effect on sore, itchy sunburnt skin. Dab it on with cotton wool as often as needed.

Sunscreens and sunblocks (*see* p.189) have different sun protection factors (SPFs) for different skin types – the fairer your skin, the higher the factor. Most people need an SPF of 15 or higher. (Much higher factors may be needed at high altitudes, when skiing, for example.) Use a sunscreen even in the shade and on cloudy days. Apply sunscreen 30 minutes before you go outside; reapply every 2 hours and each time after you have been swimming. Use a total sunblock with zinc oxide or titanium dioxide if you have very fair skin and for all children.

PREVENTION

Safety in the sun The effects of the sun on your skin don't always show straight away, so you may not realize you are burning. The following measures will help protect you from sunburn.

- Whenever your skin is exposed to the sun, use sunscreen or sunblock (*see* DRUG REMEDIES, above).
- Don't go out in summer sunshine when it is at its strongest, between 11am and 3pm.
- Don't use sunbeds.
- Be especially careful when you are close to water or snow because the reflected sunlight increases the likelihood of you getting sunburnt.
- Keep babies out of the sun completely. Use a sunshade or sit them in the shade.
- Wear loose, lightweight trousers and tops with sleeves, and also a hat, if you are out in the sun for long periods. Some clothes are now labelled with an ultraviolet protection factor (UPF), which indicates how effective they are at blocking the sun's rays.

Sun protection
Choose a hat that shades your child's face and neck and apply sunscreen to skin exposed to the sun.

Ringworm

Ringworm produces round, red, itchy, scaly patches on your skin that enlarge over a week or so to form raised red rings. It can occur anywhere, but if it affects the scalp, it also causes broken-off hairs and hair loss. Ringworm isn't caused by a worm – it is a fungal infection caught by direct contact with an infected person or pet, or from contaminated items such as towels and hairbrushes.

 See also Athlete's foot and jock itch, p.44.

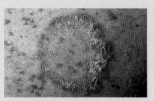
Patch of ringworm on the skin

 ## See your doctor first

Make an appointment to see your doctor if:

● You have many patches of ringworm or you have ringworm of the scalp

What you can do yourself

You may be able to clear up ringworm yourself using the following measures. Otherwise, use them with treatment that your doctor prescribes.

 ● If you have only a small area of ringworm, try an antifungal cream (*see* DRUG REMEDIES, right). Wash your hands thoroughly after touching the patches.

 ● Keep your skin clean and dry and try not to scratch. An oatmeal bath oil may help to soothe itching (*see* NATURAL REMEDIES, right).

● To prevent the infection spreading to others or reinfecting yourself, wash clothes, bed linen, and towels that you have worn or used recently. If you have scalp ringworm, also wash brushes, combs, and hats after each use.

● Don't touch animals that show signs of infection, such as hair loss. If you suspect your pet has ringworm, make sure it has veterinary treatment.

● If you have scalp ringworm, use a mild shampoo such as baby shampoo, and wash and dry your hair gently without using a hairdryer. Don't use gels, mousses, or other hair products on your hair.

● You don't need to stay away from other people but avoid contact sports until you have had at least 4 days of antifungal treatment.

 ### DRUG REMEDIES

Antifungal creams (*see* ANTIFUNGAL DRUGS, p.178) can be used to treat small areas of ringworm if you are not already using a drug or cream prescribed by your doctor. Apply the cream thinly and evenly as directed, usually 2–3 times a day, avoiding your lips and areas close to your eyes. The infection should begin to clear up within a week, although it may take several weeks to disappear. Continue using the cream for several days after your skin has started to look healthy again.

 ### NATURAL REMEDIES

Oatmeal bath oils (*see* OATMEAL PRODUCTS, p.186) can help to relieve itching. Relax in the bath for 10–20 minutes. Make sure you dry yourself thoroughly afterwards, because fungal infections thrive on warm, damp skin.

 ## Seek further medical advice

Arrange to see your doctor if:

● The patches have not started responding to treatment within a week
● Your skin is red and the patches are oozing and sore
● You have a large swelling on your scalp that is oozing pus and shedding hair

Dandruff

In this harmless but sometimes embarrassing condition, excessive amounts of skin cells flake off the scalp. They show up as white flakes in your hair, and on your shoulders if you wear dark clothes. Your scalp may also be itchy and red, and your eyelids, nose, and forehead may be affected. Dandruff is usually associated with the growth of a yeast-like fungus on the scalp, or it can be a mild form of seborrhoeic dermatitis – a scaly, itchy rash that can also affect the eyelids. Dandruff is more common in men and may be made worse by stress, illness, and some hair products. Scaly, flaking skin on a baby's scalp is known as cradle cap.

 See also Itchy eyes, p.56; Cradle cap, p.151.

What you can do yourself

Dandruff can usually be controlled with the treatments below. You may need to repeat them occasionally, because the condition tends to recur.

● Use an anti-dandruff shampoo (*see* DRUG REMEDIES, right) and wash your hair in warm rather than hot water. Massage the shampoo into your scalp and make sure you leave it on long enough to work – generally about 3–5 minutes. Rinse thoroughly afterwards.

● Keep using the brand of anti-dandruff shampoo that you find works for you. If you develop itchiness or a rash, however, stop using the shampoo immediately and try switching to one with a different active ingredient.

● Don't blow-dry your hair because it may aggravate the dandruff.

● Avoid alcohol-based hair products such as hair sprays, which tend to dry out the scalp, and mousses, gels, and dyes, which may increase irritation and make dandruff worse.

● Treat itchy, flaky skin on your eyelids (blepharitis) with a special cleaning regime (*see* PRACTICAL TECHNIQUE: CLEANING YOUR EYELIDS, p.56).

DRUG REMEDIES

Anti-dandruff shampoos (*see* p.177) should clear up your dandruff within a few weeks. Follow the instructions carefully because different brands have different treatment advice. Shampoos may contain pyrithione zinc, selenium sulphide, or ketoconazole, which is particularly effective. Alternatively, use a shampoo that contains coal tar, or coal tar and salicylic acid.

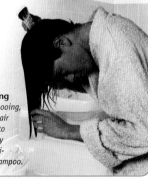

Shampooing
After shampooing, rinse your hair thoroughly to remove every trace of anti-dandruff shampoo.

Seek medical advice

Arrange to see your doctor if:

● The dandruff does not clear up after you have been using these home treatments
● You develop sensitivity to an anti-dandruff shampoo that persists for more than a few days
● Your scalp becomes red and develops sore patches or crusts

Head lice

Head lice are grey-brown insects about the size of a sesame seed that live on or close to the scalp. They lay eggs that hatch into more lice, and the oval off-white egg cases (nits) remain glued to the bases of hairs. They look like dandruff but can't be brushed off. Because head lice are easily passed on by close contact they can affect anyone, but are more common in children. You may see your child scratching his or her head, although itching may not develop until some time after infection.

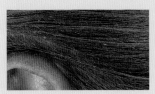
Nits in hair

 ## See your doctor first

Make an appointment to see your doctor if you aren't sure whether you have lice, or if you have lice but don't know which treatment to use.

What you can do yourself

You can treat head lice yourself, but you only need to do so if you find live lice in the hair.

 ● To detect head lice, use detection combing (*see* PRACTICAL TECHNIQUE, right). If you find lice, check family members and tell anyone who has had close contact with you or your child in the previous 4–6 weeks so they can be treated if necessary.

 ● Apply a head lice lotion to kill the lice (*see* DRUG REMEDIES, right). Shampoos are also available, but are less effective than lotions.

● If you are treating a baby under 6 months old, you should not use head lice lotions. Instead, you can use repeated detection combing (*see* PRACTICAL TECHNIQUE, right), which is also an option if you prefer not to use chemical treatments.

● Head lice die quickly once they leave the scalp but, as a precaution, wash brushes, combs, towels, and pillowcases, and don't share hats, scarves, brushes, and combs with anyone else.

 ## Seek further medical advice

Arrange to see your doctor if:

● You find live lice 2 or 3 days after the second application of a head lice lotion or after combing regularly for 2 weeks

 ### PRACTICAL TECHNIQUE

Detection combing It is difficult to find lice by just looking in the hair, so use the following process. It takes about 15–30 minutes.

● Shampoo and rinse your hair and apply a generous amount of conditioner. Comb with an ordinary comb.
● Insert a detection comb at the hair roots, with the teeth flat against the scalp. Draw it up to the hair tips.
● Check the comb after each stroke, and remove any lice by wiping it on a tissue.
● Make sure you cover the entire head, combing over a white towel so you can see any lice that fall.
● If you find lice, rinse your hair, let it dry, and apply a head lice lotion. Alternatively, rinse and repeat combing. Repeat 3 more times at 4-day intervals. If you find live lice in a subsequent session, repeat combing 3 more times, at 4-day intervals, until none are seen.

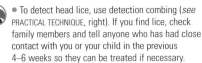

Combing method
Work backwards and forwards and from side to side over the whole head.

 ### DRUG REMEDIES

Head lice lotions (*see* p.188) contain an insecticide (malathion, permethrin, or phenothrin) or dimeticone. Alcohol-based lotions are not advised for people with asthma or eczema or for young children. Normally, you rub the lotion into the hair and scalp and leave it on overnight. You then shampoo your hair and comb out the dead lice. Reapply the lotion after 7 days.

Unwanted or ingrowing hair

Excessive hair growth (hirsutism) can affect both sexes, but is usually only a problem for women. Some women are naturally more hairy than others and may have unwanted hair on their face, and hair growing thickly on their arms, pubic area, abdomen, and thighs. Excessive hair growth can also occur during pregnancy and after the menopause. More rarely, it is due to an underlying illness or a drug. Ingrowing hairs are often caused by hair-removal methods; as the hair grows again, it curls back into the skin, causing inflammation.

 ## See your doctor first

Make an appointment to see your doctor if:

● You have noticed a recent increase in facial or body hair, and/or you have other symptoms such as irregular or absent periods, deepening of the voice, and weight increase
● You think that the hair growth may be due to a prescribed medication

What you can do yourself

If you are concerned about excess hair, try the following cosmetic measures.

 ● Use a hair-bleaching cream to lighten hair on your face (*see* DRUG REMEDIES, right).

● Pluck with tweezers to remove stray hairs under your nose and on your chin.

 ● Shaving is better for larger areas such as the legs. You can use an electric shaver or wet razor, which gives a closer shave. You will need to shave daily to avoid stubble. Shaving does not cause hair to grow back more thickly. Alternatively, use a hair removal product (*see* DRUG REMEDIES, right).

 ● Waxing is effective (*see* PRACTICAL TECHNIQUE, right) because hairs are pulled out at the root, and take up to 4 weeks to grow back. However, if you find waxing difficult, consult a beauty therapist.

 ● Ingrowing hairs usually dislodge themselves if you leave them to grow out. If not, try to lift out the end of the hair with a needle that has been sterilized under a flame, or dissolve the hair with a hair removal product (*see* DRUG REMEDIES, right). Don't shave until any inflammation has gone.

 ### DRUG REMEDIES

Hair bleaches (*see* p.183) lighten facial hair and make it less noticeable against fair skin, but they are not so suitable for darker skins.

Hair removal products (*see* p.183) include fast-acting creams and mousses that dissolve hair roots. Waxes pull out hair. Test products on a small area of skin first in case of a reaction.

 ### PRACTICAL TECHNIQUE

Waxing Before waxing, hairs need to be at least 5 mm (¼in) long and your skin clean, dry, and free of creams and oils. Take care if you have to heat the wax; very hot wax can burn your skin.

1 *Apply a thin layer of wax paste on a small section of the area to be treated, in the direction of hair growth.*

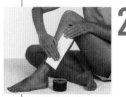

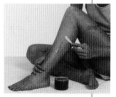

2 *Place a fabric strip over the area and smooth it down. Holding the skin taut, pull off the strip against the direction of hair growth in one swift movement.*

3 *Continue until all the unwanted hair is removed, going back over areas of stubborn hairs. Apply an unperfumed moisturizing cream afterwards. Avoid bathing or swimming until any redness has disappeared.*

Hair thinning and hair loss

Temporary hair loss often occurs after an illness or period of stress, or because of a skin infection such as ringworm. Chemical hair treatments and hairstyles and hats that pull on the hair can contribute to the problem. Some drugs and long-term illnesses cause hair loss, and women may lose hair temporarily after childbirth. Permanent hair loss is usually hereditary and can begin to affect men as early as in their twenties. Women who inherit the trait develop thin hair later in life but do not usually become bald.

➡ *See also* Ringworm, p.48.

 ## See your doctor first

Make an appointment to see your doctor if:

- You have been losing hair rapidly or in patches in recent weeks
- You think your hair loss may be due to a medication or an illness
- You are pulling your hair out

What you can do yourself

There is little you can do to prevent hereditary hair loss, but treatments may reverse some of its effects. For temporary hair loss, try the following to slow hair thinning and encourage regrowth.

- Fad diets and crash diets may contribute to hair loss. Make sure you include plenty of protein and iron in your diet (*see* NATURAL REMEDIES, right).

- Avoid using hair dyes and treatments to perm or straighten your hair. They contain chemicals that may make hair brittle and liable to break at the roots.

- Don't wear your hair in a style that pulls on your scalp, or wear a cap or hat continuously unless you have to wear headgear for your work.

- Let your hair dry naturally if possible, rather than using a hairdryer. Don't pull on your hair with a brush or comb when it is wet.

- If your hair is thinning, a good haircut can make a difference. Short, blunt cuts can make hair appear thicker. Some men prefer to cut their hair very short, or shave it off, to disguise a receding hairline.

- If you are in the early stages of hereditary hair loss, you can try a preparation containing minoxidil that may restore hair (*see* DRUG REMEDIES, right).

 ### NATURAL REMEDIES

Protein and iron Protein is essential for building and repairing tissues in the body, including hair. Make sure about one sixth of your total calorie intake is made up of foods such as meat, fish, cheese, and nuts. Iron also helps maintain healthy hair, so eat plenty of iron-rich foods such as cereals, beans, fish, poultry, meat, and leafy green vegetables.

 ### DRUG REMEDIES

Minoxidil preparations (*see* p.185) can slow down or prevent hereditary hair loss in a proportion of men and women. The treatment is applied twice daily and needs to be used continually, as its effect starts to wear off as soon as it is stopped. You may have to wait for up to a year before you notice any improvement. Ask your pharmacist for advice.

Using minoxidil
Apply the lotion to areas of hair loss using an applicator and spread it with your fingertips.

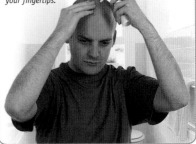

Disfigured or brittle nails

The most common cause of disfigured nails is a fungal infection. This usually affects toenails, particularly if your feet sweat a lot or you do not dry them properly after washing, although fingernails can also be infected if moisture gets trapped under artificial nails. The nail becomes thickened, crumbly, and white or yellow, and may grow misshapen or separate from the nail bed. Other nail problems include dry, hard, and brittle nails that are prone to splitting; white patches on the nails due to minor injuries; and fine vertical ridges on the nails, which are common in older people. In a few cases, nail changes indicate an underlying illness.

 See also Ingrowing toenail, p.55.

 ## See your doctor first

Make an appointment to see your doctor if:

● You have a fungal infection of the nails
● You develop abnormalities such as curved or clubbed nails or pits on the nail surfaces

What you can do yourself

Use the following tips for fragile, brittle nails and to treat a fungal infection, alongside treatment prescribed by your doctor.

● Wash your hands after touching an infected nail. If your toenails are affected, don't walk barefoot around swimming pools, showers, and locker rooms; you may pass the infection on to others.

● Wear cotton socks rather than those made of synthetic fibres and change socks, stockings, or tights daily. Wear properly fitting shoes, made from natural materials that do not trap moisture. If your feet sweat, take your shoes off during the day, if possible, or wear open-toed sandals.

 ● Practise good nail care to improve dry, brittle fingernails (*see* PRACTICAL TECHNIQUE, right).

● Wear cotton-lined rubber gloves to protect your hands when doing chores such as washing up or using household cleaning products.

● Try painting on a cosmetic nail hardener once a week. Don't wear artificial nails or nail varnish.

● Very occasionally, buff vertical ridges on nails with a fine emery board to smooth them out. Take care not to buff too much or you may thin the nail.

 PRACTICAL TECHNIQUE

Nail care This nail-care regime will help to keep your nails strong and healthy and reduce brittleness or splitting.

1 Trim your nails regularly so that they are square at the sides and slightly rounded on the top. Trim hard or brittle nails after a bath or soak them in water.

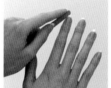

2 File your nails in one direction only, using gentle strokes from the side of the nail to its tip. Using a "sawing" motion with the file weakens the nail.

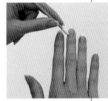

3 Don't have your cuticles removed during manicures; instead, soak your fingernails in warm water, then push the cuticles back gently with an orange stick.

4 At bedtime, rub a moisturizer into the cuticles and skin around the nails. Apply a moisturizer afterwards whenever you wash your hands.

Seek further medical advice

See your doctor if your nail problems persist or if you develop any unexplained nail symptoms.

Nailbiting

Many children and adolescents chew or bite on their fingernails, but most grow out of the habit eventually. Some people, however, continue to bite their nails in adult life, and the habit can be hard to break. You may find you bite your nails inadvertently when you are bored, or as a coping mechanism during times of stress or anxiety. Apart from being socially unappealing, nailbiting transfers germs between your hands and your mouth and, if you chew the skin around your nails as well, it becomes susceptible to infections. You may also be ashamed of the appearance of your nails, particularly if biting makes them rough, torn, or split.

 ## See your doctor first

Make an appointment to see your doctor if:

- You or your child show other signs of anxiety such as hair-pulling, or difficulty sleeping

What you can do yourself

Once you or your child have decided to stop nailbiting, take these steps to help break the habit.

- Sit in front of a mirror and watch yourself biting your nails to see how unappealing it looks.

- Cut your nails short, and smooth them with a fine emery board so there are no ragged edges to chew. Put adhesive plasters around the tops of your fingers to stop yourself chewing loose bits of skin.

- Be aware of the times when you bite your nails and try to occupy your hands by fiddling with a pen, worry beads, or a piece of modelling clay.

- Chew sugar-free gum instead of your nails.

 - Paint an anti-nailbiting lotion on your nails (see DRUG REMEDIES, right).

- Reward yourself when your nails begin to look better. For example, have a professional manicure.

- Try having artificial nails fitted. They last for about 2 weeks, which may be long enough for you to break your nailbiting habit.

- Don't make your child feel guilty about nailbiting. Try to find out if anything is causing anxiety and if there is something you can do to help.

- Use a star chart with your child. Reward each nailbiting-free day with a stick-on star and buy a small gift when the chart is complete.

DRUG REMEDIES

Anti-nailbiting lotions (see p.178) have an extremely bitter taste that deters nibbling and acts as a reminder every time you start to bite. Check the instructions before using on a child, and work with your child rather than forcing him or her to try one.

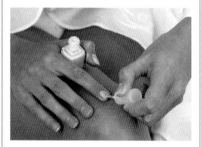

Using the lotion
Paint the lotion on like a nail varnish once a day, paying particular attention to the top edge of the nails.

 ## Seek further medical advice

Arrange to see your doctor if:

- The skin around the nails becomes red and weepy or bleeds

Ingrowing toenail

If your toe is painful, red, and swollen around the nail, the most likely cause is an ingrowing nail. Big toes are most often affected. The nail begins to grow down into the skin on either side and the area becomes inflamed. Sometimes, the skin around the nail becomes infected, in which case there may be a discharge of pus. Cutting toenails incorrectly and wearing shoes that cramp the feet are the prime causes of this problem.

 ## See your doctor first

Make an appointment to see your doctor if:

● Your toenail is inflamed and infected
● You have diabetes or poor circulation

What you can do yourself

In the early stages, when your toe is only slightly inflamed, you can treat it with the following measures. They may be enough to stop the problem getting worse.

● Soak your foot twice a day for about 10 minutes in a bowl of warm water into which you have added 2–3 tablespoonfuls of salt. Put on a dry dressing to protect the toe. Wear open-toed sandals.

● Don't cut the nail until it has fully recovered.

● Don't use nail varnish or nail varnish remover on the nail while it is inflamed.

PREVENTION

Preventing ingrowing nails The simplest way to prevent ingrowing toenails is to take good care of your feet.

● Wash your feet every day and dry them carefully.
● Don't wear shoes that squeeze or press on your toes. Avoid pointed styles and high heels.
● Change your socks, tights, or stockings daily and wear cotton socks rather than synthetics. Open-toed tights and stockings are available in some shops.
 ● Make sure you cut your toenails correctly (*see* PRACTICAL TECHNIQUE, right).

PRACTICAL TECHNIQUE

How to cut toenails Adopt this nail-cutting routine to help prevent ingrowing toenails. If you are elderly, or if you have diabetes or poor vision, seek specialist advice about nail care.

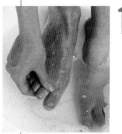

1 Soften your toenails before you trim them by soaking them for 10 minutes in a bowl of warm water or in the bath. This will make them easier to cut, especially if they are tough or thick.

2 Use sharp nail scissors or clippers to cut your toenails straight across. Shape them so that they are rounded slightly at the tip, but don't cut into the corners as this encourages them to grow inwards. Smooth the nail edges with a fine-textured file.

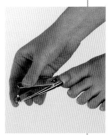

3 If a toenail is already growing into the skin, don't dig the scissors or clippers into the corner of the nail or try to push anything under the affected nail.

 ## Seek further medical advice

Arrange to see your doctor if:

● Your toe is getting worse or is not getting better after a few days of home treatment

EYE AND EAR PROBLEMS

Itchy eyes

Itchy eyes often look red, and there may also be irritation and a burning feeling. You may want to rub them continually. Anything that irritates the eyes, such as smoky atmospheres, dust, or infection, can produce itching, as can allergies such as hay fever or reactions to chlorinated swimming pools, cosmetics, or eye drops. Sometimes, the edges of the eyelids can become infected. This condition, called blepharitis, results in sore, dry eyes with crusts on the eyelashes. Blepharitis is more common in people who have skin conditions such as dandruff. You may also develop itchy eyes occasionally if you wear contact lenses.

See also Dandruff, p.49; Dry eyes, opposite page; Conjunctivitis, p.58; Contact lens problems, p.60.

See your doctor first

Make an appointment to see your doctor to establish the cause of itchy eyes.

What you can do yourself

The following steps can help relieve the problem or be used with any treatment from your doctor.

- Avoid rubbing your eyes, as this can aggravate itching and can spread an infection.

- To help soothe allergic itching and irritation, use a cold compress. Soak a clean cloth (or cotton-wool pads) in cold water, wring it out, and lay it gently on your eyes for a few minutes. Repeat as needed, using a clean cloth or pads each time.

- Use artificial tears to help soothe itching due to allergies or to irritants such as dust and smoke (*see* DRUG REMEDIES, right).

- To find out if itching is caused by sensitivity to cosmetics, soap, or face or hair products, stop using them, then reintroduce items one by one to see if the problem returns. Throw away old eye make-up; don't keep mascara for more than 6 months.

- If you have inflamed eyelids and crusty lashes, treat them with an eyelid-cleaning regime (*see* PRACTICAL TECHNIQUE, right).

DRUG REMEDIES

Artificial tears are available as drops containing hypromellose or gels containing carbomers (*see* EYE LUBRICANTS, p.181). Don't wear contact lenses while you are using these products.

PRACTICAL TECHNIQUE

Cleaning your eyelids Unless your doctor advises otherwise, try the following steps to help control blepharitis.

- Soak a clean face cloth in warm water, wring it out, then gently press it on your closed eyelid for about 5 minutes. This will soften and loosen any crusts.
- Mix a little water with an equal amount of baby shampoo. Dip a cotton-wool bud in the mixture, squeeze it out, and roll it along the edge of each eyelid to clean off debris and crusts. Rinse the eyelids with water, and dab them dry with a clean towel.
- Repeat, using a clean cloth, for the other eye.
- Clean your eyelids each morning and bedtime until they improve, then once daily to prevent a recurrence.

Seek further medical advice

Arrange to see your doctor again if:

- Symptoms persist for more than 48 hours

Dry eyes

Dry eyes tend to develop when you are not producing enough tears or the tears are not lubricating the eye properly. Your eyes may feel irritated or gritty. People of any age can be affected, but older people, particularly women after the menopause, are more susceptible. The problem is made worse by dry or windy weather, chlorinated swimming pools, and air conditioning or central heating. Diabetes, and certain medications such as antihistamines, can also cause dry eyes, as can inflammation of the eyelids (blepharitis).

 See also Itchy eyes, opposite page; Conjunctivitis, p.58; Contact lens problems, p.60.

See your doctor first

Make an appointment to see your doctor to establish the cause of dry eyes.

What you can do yourself

Try the following measures to relieve the discomfort of dry eyes.

- Blink frequently, particularly when you are focusing on detailed work for long periods. Take frequent rests if you are working at a computer.

 • For occasional dryness, use artificial tears to moisten your eyes (*see* DRUG REMEDIES, right).

 • Try using a lubricating ointment to keep your eyes moist at night (*see* DRUG REMEDIES, right).

- In centrally heated rooms, increase the humidity by using a humidifier, or place a bowl of water beside a radiator to keep the air moist.

- Drink 6–8 glasses of water a day. Cut down on coffee, tea, and cola, as these drinks contain caffeine, which can dehydrate you.

- Wear goggles when swimming.

- Avoid smoky or polluted environments, which could further irritate your eyes.

- Fit side shields to your glasses, especially in windy or dry conditions.

DRUG REMEDIES

Artificial tears include drops containing hypromellose (*see* EYE LUBRICANTS, p.181), which keep the eyes moist and help to relieve itching. Gels containing substances called carbomers (*see* EYE LUBRICANTS, p.181) also keep the eyes moist and may be more convenient than drops because they do not need to be applied as often. Don't wear contact lenses while using these products.

Lubricating eye ointment (*see* EYE LUBRICANTS, p.181) is applied at bedtime to lubricate the eyes through the night. Ask your pharmacist to recommend a suitable product.

Applying eye treatments
When using any eye treatment, apply it just inside your lower eyelid. Hold the end of the nozzle or dropper away from your eye to keep it clean.

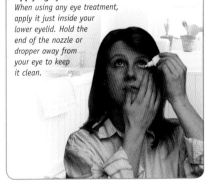

Seek further medical advice

Arrange to see your doctor again if:

- You often have dry, uncomfortable eyes
- You develop any other symptoms

Conjunctivitis

Red, itchy, gritty, and watery eyes are often due to conjunctivitis, inflammation of the membrane that covers the eye. Infectious conjunctivitis tends to start in one eye and spread to the other. Allergic conjunctivitis may be seasonal, as with hay fever, or may be due to triggers such as house dust mites and pet hairs. It can also occur as a reaction to eye make-up or chemicals in eye drops. both types may produce a discharge. In bacterial infectious conjunctivitis the discharge tends to be yellow and sticky; in other types it tends to be watery.

> ## WARNING
> Seek immediate medical help if:
> • A red eye is associated with pain, blurred or reduced vision, or sensitivity to light

See your doctor first

If you are unsure about the cause of your conjunctivitis, arrange to see your doctor.

What you can do yourself

Use the appropriate measures below to support any treatment from your doctor or to treat yourself if you are sure of the cause of your conjunctivitis.

• Avoid wearing contact lenses if you have any form of conjunctivitis until you have been free of symptoms for at least 2 days or for 24 hours after the end of treatment.

• To avoid spreading conjunctivitis due to an infection, don't share towels, and change your towel and pillowcase every day. Try not to rub your eyes; if you do, wash your hands. Throw away eye make-up that you have been using recently.

 • If your eyes are sticky or crusty each morning, clean them gently (*see* PRACTICAL TECHNIQUE, right).

• Bathe your eyes with cool water to soothe them if you have allergic conjunctivitis. Tilt your head back and pour water into the corner of the eye, allowing it to wash over the eye. Alternatively, soak a clean cloth or cotton-wool pad in cold water, wring it out, and place it over your eyes for a few minutes. Repeat as necessary, using a clean pad each time.

 • To relieve allergic conjunctivitis, use anti-allergic or antihistamine eye drops. Chloramphenicol eye drops or ointment can be used to treat bacterial conjunctivitis (*see* DRUG REMEDIES, right).

PRACTICAL TECHNIQUE

Cleaning sticky eyes Treat one eye at a time to avoid spreading infection to the other eye.

• Use a clean cotton-wool ball dipped in warm water and, with the eye closed, gently wipe along your eyelids to remove any crusts.
• Wipe from the nose outwards or the other way round, but keep wiping in the same direction.
• Repeat using fresh cotton wool for the other eye.

DRUG REMEDIES

Anti-allergic eye drops containing sodium cromoglicate (*see* p.188) can be used in the hay-fever season and regularly at other times to prevent symptoms due to house dust mites or pet hairs.

Antihistamine eye drops (*see* p.178) work quickly and are more suitable for an occasional flare-up of symptoms due to an allergic reaction.

Chloramphenicol (*see* p.179) can be used to treat conjunctivitis due to bacterial infection in those over 2 years old.

Seek further medical advice

Arrange to see your doctor if:

• Conjunctivitis is getting worse or is not responding to treatment within 48 hours

Stye

A stye is a red bump on or inside the edge of your eyelid that swells up over a few days and becomes painful. The cause is an infection at the base of an eyelash. You may find it difficult to open your eye or feel as if you have something in your eye, especially when you blink. Your eye may also be watery and sensitive to light. The stye usually comes to a head and bursts, at which point the pain subsides, although some styes disappear without coming to a head.

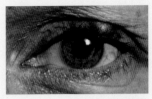

Stye on the upper eyelid

 See also Itchy eyes, p.56; Conjunctivitis, opposite page.

What you can do yourself

A stye usually clears up by itself within a few days, but the following steps will help to minimize the pain and reduce the risk of spreading the infection.

- Don't rub your eye or squeeze the stye to release pus. Put a warm compress on it to bring it to a head (*see* PRACTICAL TECHNIQUE, right).

- Once the stye has burst, bathe your eyelid with warm water, then keep your eye clean and dry.

- Wash your hands regularly and avoid rubbing or touching the affected eye.

- Don't use eye make-up on the affected eye.

- Don't wear contact lenses while you have a stye.

Seek medical advice

Arrange to see your doctor if:

- The stye hasn't healed, either on its own or with treatment, within a week
- The stye begins to spread to the skin on the surrounding eyelid
- You are getting recurrent styes

PRACTICAL TECHNIQUE

Using a warm compress Soak a cotton-wool pad or clean cloth in warm to hand-hot water, then squeeze it out and place it on your eyelid. Keep reapplying it for 10–15 minutes, rewarming the pad when it cools down. Repeat several times a day until the stye bursts.

Applying a compress
Use a clean pad for each session and keep rewarming it before holding it gently against your eyelid.

PREVENTION

Preventing styes If you are prone to styes, use these hygiene measures to help prevent them.

- Wash your hands regularly and avoid touching your eyes. Always use your own face cloth and towel.
- Throw away old eye make-up, particularly liquids such as mascaras. Don't share make-up with other people. Remove make-up before you go to bed.
- If you use non-disposable contact lenses, be particularly careful about cleaning and storing them.

Contact lens problems

The most common causes of contact lens problems are lenses that fit badly, poor lens hygiene, sensitivity to cleaning solutions, and dusty, windy environments. If you wear lenses for too long, or get a piece of grit or dirt trapped under the lens, your eyes may become irritated, red, and watery. Sometimes a lens slips under the eyelid and needs to be retrieved and repositioned.

 See also Dry eyes, p.57.

> **WARNING**
>
> Seek immediate medical help if:
> - You have pain, blurred or reduced vision, or extreme sensitivity to light
> - Your eye is very red

What you can do yourself

The following steps will help to reduce the risk of eye problems when you use contact lenses.

- If your eyes are irritated, take your contact lenses out for an hour or two to see if the symptoms ease. If they recur when you put the lenses back in, consult your optometrist or doctor.

- Try using lubricating eye drops formulated for contact lens wearers (*see* DRUG REMEDIES, right).

- Unless you use continuous-wear lenses, don't wear your lenses for longer than the period of time advised by your optometrist. If this is unavoidable, take them out from time to time to give your eyes a rest. Always remove lenses before going to bed, having a nap, or swimming, bathing, or showering.

- Before handling lenses, wash your hands using an antibacterial or unperfumed soap and rinse them thoroughly. Clean and rinse reusable lenses every time you remove them using approved cleaners and storage solutions. Clean the lens case and air dry it too. Never lick your lenses or use water to wet them.

- Ask your optometrist about using disposable contact lenses, which are worn for just one day and discarded. They don't need to be cleaned and sterilized and may be less likely to irritate your eyes.

- Take care with make-up. Apply it after you put your lenses in, and don't use powder eye shadow or loose powder. Keep hairspray away from your eyes.

- Contact lenses can't really get "lost" in the eye, but sometimes a lens slips under the eyelid. Try this technique to get the lens back into position (*see* PRACTICAL TECHNIQUE, right).

DRUG REMEDIES

Eye drops containing sodium chloride (*see* EYE LUBRICANTS, p.181) lubricate the eye and make it easier to insert and remove lenses. Don't use other types of eye drops without seeking advice from your pharmacist because some may damage your lenses.

PRACTICAL TECHNIQUE

If a lens has slipped under your eyelid, the following steps will help you retrieve it.

1 *First, squeeze 1–2 lubricating eye drops into your eye. If your eye is dry, using drops may be enough to help the lens float back into its correct position.*

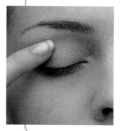

2 *If this doesn't work, close your eye, then guide the lens back into position by pressing lightly on your eyelid with one finger. This should encourage the lens to slide back down over the front of your eye.*

Seek medical advice

See your doctor or optometrist promptly if:

- Eye irritation continues or there is a discharge
- You develop any new eye problems

Foreign object in the eye

If you get something in your eye, it can cause irritation, redness, watering, and blurred vision. In many instances, the foreign object is something tiny, such as an eyelash or a speck of dust or grit, and will wash out automatically as you blink and produce tears. If it remains floating on the white of your eye and you are sure there is no other injury, you can usually remove it yourself or get someone to remove it for you.

WARNING

Seek immediate medical attention if:
● An object sticks on or in the eye, or rests on the iris
● You think something entered your eye while you were using a power tool, or hammering or chiselling

What you can do yourself

Take the following steps to remove a speck of dust or debris on the white of an eye.

● Don't rub the affected eye. Wash your hands thoroughly. If you are wearing contact lenses, remove them straight away.

● If you are treating someone else, sit the person in a well-lit place and check the eye for specks by gently pulling down the lower eyelid and asking him or her to look upwards and then to the right and to the left. Repeat the procedure for the upper eyelid, pulling the eyelid up and asking the person to look down, right, and left. To check your own eye, sit in front of a mirror and pull your lower lid down and then the upper lid up.

 ● If you do find a speck of debris on the white of the eye, try flushing the eye with water (*see* PRACTICAL TECHNIQUE, right).

● If the speck has not been flushed out, try to lift it off the eye by lightly touching it with the edge of a clean, dampened handkerchief or tissue.

● If the speck is under the upper eyelid, grasp the upper lashes and pull the upper eyelid over the lower one to brush it out of the eye.

Seek medical advice

Arrange immediate medical help if:

● A foreign object cannot be removed easily
● You suffer pain, redness, extreme sensitivity to light, or blurred vision after you have removed a particle from your eye

PRACTICAL TECHNIQUE

Flushing out a foreign object

Use this procedure to flush a speck of debris out of your own or another person's eye.

● Treat another person's eye by putting a towel round his or her shoulders to catch run-off. Tilt the head to one side so that the affected eye is lower. Pour the water into the uppermost corner of the eye and let it drain out of the other side.
● Treat your own eye by filling a small glass, or eyebath if you have one, with water. Put a towel round your shoulders to catch run-off. Rest the rim of the glass or eye bath on the bone of the lower part of your eye socket. Keeping your eye open, tip your head back and pour in water to wash out the speck.

Flushing your eye
Pour the water directly into your eye, letting it drain freely on to the towel.

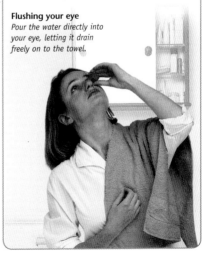

Black eye

A black eye is a bruise that develops around the eye, usually as a result of a direct blow to the eye. You may also get a black eye with other facial injuries because the skin around the eyes is delicate and easily bruised. Swelling, tenderness, and bleeding under the skin usually develop shortly after the injury. Later, the eyelids and surrounding area turn bluish-black, and gradually fade to purple and then yellow as the bruise heals. Most black eyes disappear within 10–14 days.

> **WARNING**
>
> Seek medical help immediately if:
> - You cannot see clearly and/or have blurred or double vision
> - Your eye or eyelid is injured
> - You lost consciousness, even for a short time

 ## See your doctor first

Arrange to see your doctor urgently if:

- You are not certain how the black eye was caused or are concerned in any way about the condition of your eye

What you can do yourself

For a black eye caused by a minor injury, start using these home treatments as soon as possible to minimize bruising and discomfort.

 - Apply an icepack to the eye to reduce swelling and bleeding (see PRACTICAL TECHNIQUE, right).

- Keep your head raised on pillows at night to reduce the swelling.

- If necessary, take a painkiller (see DRUG REMEDIES, right) to relieve discomfort.

- Avoid contact sports until your eye has healed.

- Try not to blow your nose hard because it increases blood flow to the face and makes swelling around the eye worse.

 ## Seek further medical advice

Arrange to see your doctor if:

- The black eye is not healing after a few days, becomes hot and swollen, or leaks pus
- There is any alteration in your vision
- You have persistent pain or headaches

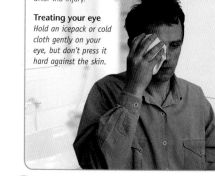

PRACTICAL TECHNIQUE

Applying an icepack Put something cold on a black eye as soon as possible to reduce swelling and bleeding under the skin.

- Use a bag of frozen peas or crushed ice wrapped in a wet towel, or a cloth soaked in cold water and wrung out. (If none are available, use a can of cold drink held lightly to the edge of the bruised area.)
- Hold the icepack or cloth for 10–15 minutes without applying direct pressure to the eye.
- Reapply up to 8 times a day for the first 24–48 hours after the injury.

Treating your eye
Hold an icepack or cold cloth gently on your eye, but don't press it hard against the skin.

DRUG REMEDIES

Painkillers Paracetamol (see p.187) or ibuprofen (see p.184) will reduce the discomfort of a black eye. Avoid aspirin because it may prolong the bleeding that causes a black eye.

Earwax

Normally, earwax is produced in small amounts that protect the ear canal and disperse naturally. But if too much wax is produced, it can build up, become hard and dry, and block your ear canal. Using a cotton bud to clean the ears can cause wax to become impacted and contribute to blockages. A build-up of wax can cause hearing loss, discomfort, and a feeling of fullness in the ear. You may also notice itching, ringing (tinnitus), or dizziness. Wax build-up is more common in elderly people and in people who wear hearing aids.

 See also Earache, p.64; Tinnitus, p.67.

See your doctor first

Arrange to see your doctor to confirm that there is a build-up of earwax, especially if you have had previous ear problems.

What you can do yourself

You only need to treat earwax if it is causing problems. You may be able to clear a build-up completely with the following measures. If you need to have your ears syringed by a doctor, these steps will also help to soften wax beforehand.

● Never use cotton buds or push anything into your ear to clear wax. Apart from pushing wax further into the ear canal, you may damage the ear canal lining, causing irritation and infection, or even damage the eardrum itself.

 ● Treat your ears with something that will soften the wax. Try using olive oil, almond oil, or sodium bicarbonate drops (*see* PRACTICAL TECHNIQUE, right).

 ● If the above are not effective, try ear drops containing a wax solvent (*see* DRUG REMEDIES, right).

Seek further medical advice

Arrange to see your doctor if:

● Your ear still feels as if it is blocked after you have tried self-help measures
● You develop earache or a discharge of pus

PRACTICAL TECHNIQUE

Softening wax in your ear You can buy olive oil, almond oil, or sodium bicarbonate drops from your pharmacist (*see* EAR WAX DROPS, p.181). Ask for a dropper if one is not supplied. If both ears are blocked, wait until one ear has cleared before treating the other, because the blockage may worsen temporarily as the wax softens.

● Allow half an hour for the olive or almond oil to warm to room temperature, or speed up the process by standing the bottle in warm water. You can use sodium bicarbonate drops straight away.
● Lying with the blocked ear upwards, use a dropper to put 3–4 drops into the ear canal. Wait 10 minutes for them to be absorbed, then wipe off any excess.
● Repeat the process 3 times a day for 5 days.

Warming oils
Warm the olive or almond oil slightly by standing it in a bowl of hand-hot water for 10 minutes.

DRUG REMEDIES

Solvent ear wax drops (*see* p.181) can be used but they contain chemicals such as hydrogen peroxide that sometimes irritate the ear canal. Ask your pharmacist for advice.

Earache

Pain in one or both ears and temporary hearing loss are often caused by a middle-ear infection, in which case you may also have a fever and feel generally unwell. Sometimes, the eardrum bursts as a result of increased pressure and there is a discharge from the ear. Earache can also be caused by infection in the outer ear (swimmer's ear) or be associated with a throat or sinus infection or a tooth problem. You may also get a mild earache because of a build-up of mucus in your ear after a cold; during an attack of hay fever; or from pressure changes in the ear if you travel by plane or go diving.

 See also Swimmer's ear, opposite page; Popping ears, p.66; Sinusitis, p.79; Earache (children), p.140.

 ## See your doctor first

Make an appointment to see your doctor if:

- You have severe earache, develop a fever, or have a discharge from your ear

What you can do yourself

While following your doctor's advice, there are several measures you can take to relieve earache or to treat a mild earache yourself.

 - Take painkillers to reduce the discomfort (*see* DRUG REMEDIES, right).

- Sleep with your head raised on several pillows to reduce pressure in the middle ear.

 - If your earache is due to a cold, try using decongestant nasal sprays or drops to help clear your nasal passages (*see* DRUG REMEDIES, right).

 - Apply warmth to your ear to help relieve your earache (*see* PRACTICAL TECHNIQUE, right).

- Steam inhalation (*see* PRACTICAL TECHNIQUE, p.79) can help relieve congestion in the ear, nose, and sinuses. Putting a humidifier in the room may help.

- If your eardrum bursts, there may be a discharge. Keep your ear dry and arrange to see your doctor.

Seek further medical advice

Arrange to see your doctor if:

- Your symptoms become more severe or do not subside within 24 hours of treatment

 ### DRUG REMEDIES

Painkillers Paracetamol (*see* p.187) and ibuprofen (see p.184) will reduce discomfort, and will also reduce fever if you have an ear infection.

Decongestants (*see* p.181) in the form of nasal sprays or drops can help to clear congestion in the nose, sinuses, and middle ear when you have a cold or allergy. Don't use a decongestant for more than 7 days continuously. If you use one for longer you may have a "rebound effect" with symptoms returning when you stop taking the drug.

 ### PRACTICAL TECHNIQUE

Using compresses You can make a warm compress by soaking a face cloth in warm water and squeezing it out. Hold the compress over the affected ear until the cloth cools down; then rewarm it. Alternatively, rest your ear on a heated pad or a covered hot-water bottle.

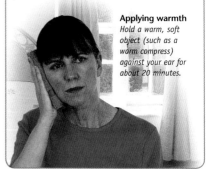

Applying warmth
Hold a warm, soft object (such as a warm compress) against your ear for about 20 minutes.

Swimmer's ear

It's not only swimmers who get swimmer's ear (otitis externa). When you shower or wash your hair, trapped moisture can carry germs into the ear canal and cause an infection; the problem can also develop after ear syringing or if you work in warm and humid environments. Your ear may feel itchy and painful (particularly when you touch or pull your earlobe) and may feel blocked. There may also be a discharge of fluid from the ear. A scratch to the delicate lining of the ear canal, or a reaction to chemicals in ear drops or hair dyes, can also cause irritation and/or infection of the ear canal.

 See also Earwax, p.63.

 ## See your doctor first

Make an appointment to see your doctor if you think you might have swimmer's ear, to confirm the diagnosis.

What you can do yourself

Dealt with promptly, swimmer's ear normally clears up within a week or two. There are several things you can do to support treatment from your doctor.

- Your ear will be itchy, but don't scratch it.

- Don't use ear drops or treatments that have not been prescribed by your doctor.

- Keep your ear as dry as possible during treatment and for several days afterwards. Take baths rather than showers. When you wash your hair, keep water out of your ears by placing pads of soft cotton wool coated with petroleum jelly inside the entrance to each ear canal. Remove the pads afterwards. Don't swim until the infection has cleared up.

 - Hold a warm, dry face cloth or a covered hot-water bottle against your ear to help relieve the pain. Taking painkillers may also help (*see* DRUG REMEDIES, right).

- If you have a discharge, place a piece of cotton wool over the outer part of your ear to absorb it. Make sure you change the cotton wool regularly. Don't try to clean your ear canal with cotton buds, while you have an ear infection or at other times. They can damage your ear.

DRUG REMEDIES

Painkillers Take paracetamol (*see* p.187) or ibuprofen (*see* p.184) to relieve any pain.

PREVENTION

Protecting your ears If you are prone to swimmer's ear, try these steps to help prevent it.

- Wear earplugs when you swim, and don't swim in polluted or dirty water.
- Always dry your ears carefully after washing your hair or showering. Tilt your head to one side and pull gently on each earlobe to help the water run out. Then use a hairdryer.
- Use unperfumed shampoos, and avoid hair dyes and styling products.

Drying safely
Use a hairdryer on a low heat and speed setting and hold it about 30 cm (12 in) from each ear.

 ## Seek further medical advice

Arrange to see your doctor again if:

- **Your symptoms get worse or have not begun to respond to treatment after 2 days**

Popping ears

The feeling of "popping ears" is common during air travel, scuba-diving, or even when you travel up or down steep hills in a car. It is due to a difference in pressure between the outside environment and your middle ear, which makes your eardrum bulge and may cause pain, a muffled feeling, ringing in your ears, and temporary hearing loss. Normally, pressures are kept equal by air flowing in and out of the middle ear via the eustachian tubes, which link the middle ear to the nose and throat, but during rapid ascent or descent the tubes are too narrow to cope. Babies and young children have short, narrow tubes and are particularly prone to popping ears. Your ears are also more likely to pop if you have a blocked nose.

What you can do yourself

There are several steps that you can take to help equalize the pressure in your ears. The discomfort of popping ears usually disappears 3–5 hours after air pressure has stabilized.

- On a plane, chew gum or suck boiled sweets when you are ascending or descending rapidly.
- Swallowing frequently with your mouth open or yawning helps to equalize the pressure.
- You can use a simple technique to unblock your ears (*see* PRACTICAL TECHNIQUE, right).
- If you are travelling with a baby, try breastfeeding or bottle-feeding while the plane is ascending or descending, or let your baby suck a dummy. Give your baby plenty of fluids to drink during travel.
- If you are particularly susceptible to popping ears, take a decongestant before you travel (*see* DRUG REMEDIES, right).
- If you have a cold, an ear infection, or sinusitis, try to avoid air travel. If you must fly, use a decongestant. If you have hay fever when you fly, take an antihistamine (*see* DRUG REMEDIES, right). Don't scuba-dive if you have any of these conditions.

Seek medical advice

Arrange to see your doctor if:

- Your ears are very painful.
- Symptoms don't subside within 3–5 hours of returning to normal air pressure
- You have a discharge from your ear
- You have persistent hearing loss

PRACTICAL TECHNIQUE

Unblocking your ears Try the following action to relieve discomfort and unblock your ears. You may need to do this several times during ascent or descent.

- Begin by firmly pinching both of your nostrils closed with your index finger and thumb.
- Breathe in through your mouth. Then close your mouth, hold your nose tightly, and gently blow into your nostrils until your ears pop.

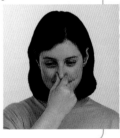

Blowing into your nostrils
Be careful not to blow too hard as you could damage your eardrums.

DRUG REMEDIES

Decongestants (*see* p.180), available as drops, sprays, and tablets, shrink the membranes lining the nasal passages. When you fly, use a decongestant an hour before you take off, and repeat as necessary, following the instructions supplied with the product.

Antihistamines (*see* p.178) will relieve a blocked or runny nose caused by hay fever for the duration of your flight. Take a non-sedative antihistamine before travelling. Repeat as necessary, according to the instructions on the pack.

Tinnitus

If you suffer from tinnitus, you experience ringing, buzzing, or hissing noises that seem to be generated inside your ears or head with no external source for the sound. The noises, which may be continuous or may come and go, can affect sleep and concentration, and may make you depressed and anxious over time. Tinnitus is often linked to hearing loss, particularly in later life, or to repeated exposure to loud noise. Stress may make the problem worse. Air travel, high blood pressure, earwax build-up, certain inner ear problems, and some medications can all contribute to tinnitus. Sometimes, however, there is no apparent cause.

 See also Earwax, p.63; **Popping ears**, opposite page.

See your doctor first

Make an appointment to see your doctor to confirm tinnitus and to find out whether a medicine you are taking, such as aspirin, is causing the problem or making it worse.

What you can do yourself

There isn't always a cure for tinnitus, but there are various things you can do that minimize its effects and make it easier to live with.

● Try using other sounds to distract you and mask the tinnitus (*see* PRACTICAL TIPS, right).

● Protect your ears with earplugs or earmuffs in noisy places or when you are using power tools such as a drill, as loud noise may make tinnitus worse.

● Cut down on caffeinated drinks such as coffee and cola. You should also avoid tonic water (which contains quinine), alcohol, and tobacco smoke. All of these substances make tinnitus worse.

● A low-salt diet may be helpful. Add less salt to your cooking and use herbs and spices instead.

● If stress makes your tinnitus worse, take regular exercise and try using measures to reduce stress in your life (*see* STRESS, pp.20–21).

● If you have persistent tinnitus, joining a support group for sufferers can be a good way to share problems and discuss solutions.

PRACTICAL TIPS

Distraction methods Some people who suffer from tinnitus find that it helps to use other sounds to mask the noises in their ears, particularly at night when there is naturally less ambient noise and the tinnituis noises may be more noticeable and may make it difficult to sleep. Often, the most effective masking sound is white noise – a hissing sound – although some people prefer identifiable sounds, such as music or talk. You may have to experiment to find the sound that works best for you. The following are suggestions you can try.

● Put a noisy fan that produces a noticeable whirring sound by your bed or on your desk.
● Use a radio that is tuned off-station to produce a hissing noise, which is similar to white noise.
● Use a personal music player to play sounds of your choice through earphones or headphones.
● Try a wearable noise generator.This resembles a hearing aid and produces a soothing "shh" sound.
● Special bedside or desktop noise generators are also available. They produce a variety of sounds, such as a waterfall or birdsong, which can be played through loudspeakers, headphones, earphones, or special speakers designed to go under a pillow.

Seek further medical advice

Arrange to see your doctor again if:

● Your tinnitus gets worse, or does not respond to the treatment advised by your doctor or to the self-help measures described above
● You also feel dizzy or sick
● You develop hearing loss

Foreign object in the ear

If something becomes lodged in your ear it can cause irritation, and can result in temporary hearing loss if it blocks your ear canal. A sharp object can damage your eardrum. Young children sometimes push small items such as beads or bits of paper into their ears. Unless you see them doing it, you may not be aware of a problem until they complain of pain in the ear, have a discharge from it, or are unable to hear properly. Adults sometimes get cotton wool stuck inside the ear canal while cleaning their ears (a practice that is not recommended). Occasionally, insects get lodged in the ears; this can be alarming, especially for a child.

 See also Earwax, p.63.

 ## See your doctor

Make an urgent appointment to see your doctor if an object does not fall out of the ear by itself or if you cannot remove an insect using the measures below.

What you can do yourself

There are limited steps that you can take to deal with an object or insect in the ear; if they don't work, see your doctor.

- Try tilting the ear downwards and shaking it gently to see if the object or insect falls out.

 • If there is an insect in the ear, try to stay calm. Tilt the affected ear upwards and wait to see if the insect crawls out by itself. If it doesn't, try floating it out with water (*see* PRACTICAL TECHNIQUE, right).

- Never try to remove something from the ear by probing with fingers, tweezers, or a cotton bud, even if you can see it. You are likely to push the object further into the ear, and may damage the lining of the ear and/or the eardrum.

 ## Seek further medical advice

Arrange to see your doctor urgently if, after removing an object:

- There is still a feeling of something in the ear
- Your hearing is impaired
- Your ear is painful or there is a discharge

 ### PRACTICAL TECHNIQUE

Removing an insect from the ear You may be able to remove an insect from the ear by floating it out. If the insect is in your own ear, get someone to help you. (Don't use water to remove anything other than an insect, because some objects may swell up and become more difficult to remove.)

- Have some tepid water ready and a dropper.
- Ask the person to lie down with the affected ear upwards and to keep very still.
- Trickle water into the ear using the dropper. This should cause the insect to float out of the ear.
- Tilt the head downwards to let any remaining water drain away.
- If the insect does not float out, don't make further attempts to remove it. Seek medical help.

Floating out an insect
A child may be frightened at the thought of having an insect in the ear, so calm him or her down first. Ask the child to lie very still while you drop water into the ear.

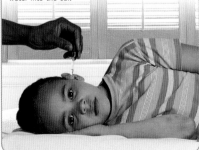

MOUTH, NOSE, AND THROAT PROBLEMS

Chapped or cracked lips

Almost everyone gets dry, chapped lips occasionally. Lips are sensitive to sunlight, and dry out easily in cold, windy weather and in centrally heated rooms. The problem is made worse if you lick your lips habitually. These same conditions can cause cracks in the skin folds at the corners of the mouth where moisture gathers. The skin may be sore, and you may have a burning sensation when you open your mouth. The area may become weepy, and a yeast infection may develop. Elderly people, particularly those who have worn-down dentures or teeth missing, are prone to the problem, as are babies who dribble or overuse a dummy. Underlying illnesses such as anaemia can contribute. An allergic reaction, for example to cosmetics, may also cause sore lips.

What you can do yourself

Just a few days of care and attention will help to improve the condition of dry, sore lips and related problems. Combine the treatment with preventive measures to protect your lips.

● If you have cracked or sore lips, put some petroleum jelly on them or try a cream or balm from your pharmacist. Before you go out in cold, dry weather, apply a moisturizing lip salve on and around your lips (*see* DRUG REMEDIES, right).

● If you suspect that your lip symptoms are an allergic reaction, throw away any toothpastes, cosmetics, and lip products that you have been using. Introduce a new toothpaste and new lip products one by one and watch for reactions.

● Avoid acidic or spicy foods or drinks that may "burn" sore skin.

● Drink plenty of water (at least 6–8 glasses a day), particularly when the central heating is on.

● Try to stop licking your lips.

● See your dentist if you have teeth problems: for example, if your dentures do not fit well.

DRUG REMEDIES

Lip creams, balms, and salves
(*see* p.185) moisturize and soothe sore, chapped lips and cracked corners of the mouth. Use a lip salve with a minimum sun protection factor (SPF) of 15 in hot sunshine and one with an SPF of 25 or higher at high altitudes. Most contain moisturizers and are water-resistant. Ask your pharmacist for advice.

Protecting your lips
Reapply lip balm or salve frequently, especially in cold, windy weather and at high altitudes.

 ## Seek medical advice

Arrange to see your doctor if:

● The area of skin becomes red and weepy and there is a discharge
● The cracked skin is getting worse or is not getting better after about 10 days
● You regularly get cracked mouth corners

Cold sore

Cold sores begin with tingling near the mouth, followed by a cluster of small, painful blisters. These sores burst and crust over, but normally heal within about 10 days. They are caused by the herpes simplex virus, which lies dormant in the body after a first infection. Triggers such as colds and flu, tiredness, stress, menstruation, cold, wind, or strong sunshine can reactivate the virus, causing another cold sore.

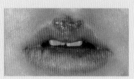

Cold sore on lip

 ### See your doctor first

Make an appointment to see your doctor promptly if you are developing a cold sore in or near your eye.

What you can do yourself

You can't get rid of the cold sore virus, but the following measures will reduce the time for which a cold sore lasts and help to prevent flare-ups.

 • Use aciclovir cream at the first sign of tingling or itching in a cold sore (see DRUG REMEDIES, right).

• As soon as you notice tingling, apply a small ice pack (a packet of frozen peas or crushed ice in a plastic bag, wrapped in a face cloth) to the area, for about 5–10 minutes every half hour.

 • Take a painkiller if you are finding your cold sore is very uncomfortable (see DRUG REMEDIES, right).

• Apply petroleum jelly to the affected area to help prevent cracking or bleeding.

• Cold sores are contagious. While you have symptoms, avoid close contact such as kissing and don't share towels, cups and glasses, or razors.

• After touching a sore, wash your hands to avoid spreading the virus. Don't pick or squeeze sores.

• If sunlight triggers cold sores, use sunscreen or a lip balm with sunscreen when you spend time in the sun (see DRUG REMEDIES, p.69).

• If stress or fatigue are triggers, get plenty of sleep, and try deep breathing and muscle relaxation exercises (see PRACTICAL TECHNIQUES, pp.20–21).

 ### DRUG REMEDIES

Painkillers such as paracetamol (see p.187) or ibuprofen (see p.184) can help to ease the discomfort of a cold sore.

Aciclovir cream (see p.177) acts against the herpes virus and can reduce the duration and severity of a cold sore. Wash your hands after applying it. If the sore has not healed after 5 days, use the cream for another 5 days.

Using aciclovir
Apply aciclovir cream thinly to the area as soon as you notice the signs that a cold sore is developing.

 ### Seek further medical advice

Arrange to see your doctor if:

• The sore is getting worse, or is not getting better after about 10 days despite treatment
• You have frequent cold sores

Mouth ulcer

Common mouth ulcers start with burning pain or soreness, then a shallow, greyish-white pit with a red border develops. The ulcers tend to recur, but are not contagious. They are more likely to develop if you are run down or stressed. Some women get them before a period. Badly fitting dentures or careless toothbrushing can also cause them. Rarely, an ulcer in the mouth may be due to cancer.

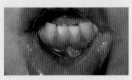

Common mouth ulcer on gum

 ## See your doctor first

Make an appointment to see your doctor if:

- You also feel sick and/or have a fever
- Many ulcers develop at the same time
- You have had a mouth ulcer for longer than 2 weeks and/or it is getting bigger

What you can do yourself

A common mouth ulcer normally disappears within a week or two without treatment, but it can be very uncomfortable. Try the following measures to reduce pain and help the ulcer heal more quickly.

- Eat soft, soothing foods, such as yoghurt, ice cream, and custard. Sip cool water or other cooling drinks through a straw.

- Avoid any food or drink that will irritate your mouth and aggravate your ulcer, such as citrus fruits and drinks; coffee; salty or spicy foods; hard, scratchy foods such as nuts, crisps, and toast; and very hot food or drinks.

- Clean your teeth using a soft toothbrush.

 - Use an antiseptic mouthwash (*see* DRUG REMEDIES, right). Alternatively, make a salt-water mouthwash by dissolving half a teaspoon of salt in 250 ml (half a pint) of warm water and use it several times a day. Swish the mouthwash around your mouth for about 30 seconds, then spit it out.

 - Apply a mouth ulcer paste containing a steroid to ease pain, aid healing, and protect your ulcer from irritants (*see* DRUG REMEDIES, right).

 - Ease pain with a mouth rinse or spray containing a painkiller, or a lozenge, gel, or spray containing a local anaesthetic (*see* DRUG REMEDIES, right).

DRUG REMEDIES

Antiseptic mouthwashes Rinsing your mouth for about 1 minute twice a day with a mouthwash containing chlorhexidine (*see* MOUTH AND THROAT TREATMENTS, p.186) reduces the risk of a secondary infection and will help your mouth ulcer to heal.

Mouth ulcer treatments (*see* p.186) include a mouth ulcer paste containing a steroid drug that reduces inflammation and helps healing. The sticky paste helps to keep the treatment in place. Apply it after a meal and at bedtime, so that it stays in contact with your ulcer for longer.

Mouth and throat treatments (*see* p.186) Rinses, sprays, or gels containing the painkiller benzydamine can help to reduce the pain and inflammation of a mouth ulcer. Speak to your pharmacist before using one to treat a child. Some products contain a local anaesthetic to numb the area and provide temporary relief; however, using an anaesthetic regularly may increase irritation.

 ## Seek further medical advice

Arrange to see your doctor if:

- You have severe pain that is not controlled by the measures described above
- You have difficulty swallowing
- The ulcer has not healed within 2 weeks and/or it is getting bigger
- You have recurrent mouth ulcers

Bad breath

Unpleasant-smelling breath, known medically as halitosis, is usually due to poor mouth hygiene. Particles of food left in the mouth and between the teeth are broken down by bacteria and cause an offensive smell. Particular foods and drinks, such as garlic and beer, can make your breath smell. Bad breath also tends to occur when your mouth is dry, and is often a problem on waking. Other possible causes include a sinus or throat infection, diabetes, lung disease, or a weight-loss diet.

What you can do yourself

The following simple measures will help you tackle bad breath. Make them part of your daily routine.

● Brush your teeth before going to bed and when you get up. Brush your tongue as well. Use a soft-bristled brush and a fluoride toothpaste, and make sure you rinse thoroughly afterwards.

● Floss your teeth once a day to remove plaque (see PRACTICAL TECHNIQUE: ORAL HYGIENE, p.74).

● If you wear dentures, take them out at night and clean them thoroughly, as recommended by your dentist. You should also clean removable braces and fixed dental appliances as advised by your orthodontist.

● Make sure you eat breakfast because it stimulates saliva, which helps to wash away bacteria that may have built up overnight. Fruit and vegetables also stimulate saliva, so include plenty of them in your daily diet.

● Take a toothbrush to work or school so you can brush after meals. If you can't clean your teeth between meals, chew sugar-free gum, which encourages saliva flow.

● Mouthwashes and breath fresheners have only a cosmetic effect but can be a useful short-term measure (see DRUG REMEDIES, right).

● Avoid spicy or strong-smelling food. When you can't avoid it, finish the meal with some fruit.

● Drink at least 6–8 glasses of water each day. Avoid alcohol, tea, and coffee; they have a dehydrating effect that can encourage bad breath.

● Don't smoke. Cigarettes are a major cause of bad breath.

DRUG REMEDIES

Mouthwashes (see MOUTH AND THROAT TREATMENTS, p.186) usually contain flavourings and extracts to freshen the breath. They may also contain antiseptics, painkillers, and/or fluoride. Don't give mouthwashes to children because they could easily swallow them.

Breath fresheners (see MOUTH AND THROAT TREATMENTS, p.186), in the form of sprays and little tablets that dissolve on the tongue, can be an effective short-term remedy for bad breath. They mask the breath with a pleasant (usually minty) smell; the effect usually lasts for about 20 minutes.

Breath freshening
Use a breath-freshener spray as a temporary measure to mask lingering smells after a spicy meal.

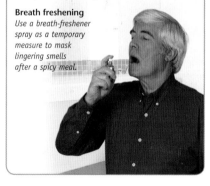

 Seek medical advice

Arrange to see your doctor if:

● You have tried the above measures for about a week and bad breath persists
● You also have toothache, or inflamed or bleeding gums
● You feel generally unwell and think this may be contributing to bad breath

Sore mouth or tongue

There are several possible causes for a sore mouth or tongue. The lining of your mouth can become irritated and inflamed by hot, spicy foods or hot drinks, or because you overuse mouthwashes, drink heavily, or smoke. Your tongue may be tender and have a smooth, red appearance, and your sense of taste may be altered. You may also get a sore mouth if you bite your tongue or cheek accidentally, or if you have rough or broken teeth or badly fitting dentures. Other causes include common mouth ulcers, gum disorders, and mouth infections such as thrush. In rare cases, a sore mouth is caused by a more serious illness.

 See also Mouth ulcer, p.71; Bleeding gums, p.74.

See your doctor first

Make an appointment to see your doctor if:

- You have signs of an infection, such as white patches inside your mouth
- You feel lethargic, are not eating well, and/or are losing weight
- Your mouth and eyes are persistently dry

What you can do yourself

Use the following home treatments to soothe an irritated mouth and tongue:

- Drink 6–8 glasses of fluid a day. Cool drinks and ice lollies are soothing. Don't drink alcohol or smoke – both can irritate your mouth.

 - Try using a homemade mouthwash (*see* NATURAL REMEDIES, right). Avoid mouthwashes that contain alcohol because they may cause further irritation.

- Don't give up cleaning your teeth, just do it gently using a very soft toothbrush.

- Eat small, frequent meals of soft foods, such as milk puddings, mashed potato and gravy, yoghurt, and custard. Avoid salty, spicy foods, coarse foods such as toast, and acidic fruit juices.

 - Try using a painkilling mouth treatment (*see* DRUG REMEDIES, right).

- If you have a dry mouth, use sugar-free chewing gum to stimulate saliva flow.

- See your dentist if you have rough or broken teeth, or if your dentures don't fit properly.

NATURAL REMEDIES

Soothing mouthwash Dissolve half a teaspoon of sodium bicarbonate (*see* p.188) or salt in 250 ml (half a pint) of warm water, and use this to rinse your mouth regularly during the day, especially after eating. Swish the mouthwash around your mouth for about 30 seconds before spitting it out.

DRUG REMEDIES

Painkilling mouth treatments (*see* MOUTH AND THROAT TREATMENTS, p.186) can help to relieve soreness. Some rinses, lozenges, and sprays reduce pain and inflammation, while others contain a local anaesthetic that numbs sore areas. However, using anaesthetic preparations regularly may increase irritation. Ask your pharmacist for advice before giving mouth treatments to a child.

Seek further medical advice

Arrange to see your doctor if:

- The soreness becomes worse, or does not subside after a few days of using the self-help measures described here

Bleeding gums

Bleeding from the gums is usually a sign of gum inflammation (gingivitis). Healthy gums are pale and firm, but diseased gums may become purplish-red, swollen, and shiny, and bleed when you brush your teeth. Your breath may smell unpleasant. The cause is usually a build-up of plaque (a deposit formed from food particles, saliva, and bacteria) at the base of the teeth due to poor oral hygiene. Bleeding gums can also be due to vigorous brushing or poorly fitting dentures. You may be prone to them during pregnancy or if you take certain drugs.

 See also Bad breath, p.72.

 ## See your dentist or doctor first

Arrange to see your dentist or doctor if:

- You have toothache or loose teeth
- You bruise easily and feel tired and weak
- You are taking a prescribed medicine, such as an anticoagulant, that may cause bleeding gums. Don't stop taking prescribed medicine without consulting your doctor

What you can do yourself

Use these measures to help your gums heal and prevent more serious damage to gums and teeth.

- If bleeding is profuse, try pressing a piece of gauze or cotton wool soaked in ice-cold water on your gums for a few minutes.

 - Practise good oral hygiene (*see* PRACTICAL TECHNIQUE, right). Brush your teeth gently using a new, soft-bristled brush, making sure you don't scratch your gums. Use dental tape or floss, or a tapered interdental brush (which looks like a tiny bottlebrush), to clean between your teeth.

- Don't use toothpicks to clean between your teeth, because they can injure your gums.

- Stop smoking, because tobacco smoke aggravates bleeding gums.

 ## Seek further medical advice

Arrange to see your dentist or doctor if:

- Your gums are still bleeding after you have tried the above measures for 7–10 days
- You have any other symptoms

 ### PRACTICAL TECHNIQUE

Oral hygiene The following oral hygiene routine helps to reduce the risk of gum disease and prevent tooth decay. Brush your teeth at least twice a day, and replace your toothbrush every 2–3 months. Clean between your teeth with dental floss or tape. There are many types available; tape may be more comfortable for your gums.

1 *Brush your teeth before going to bed and when you get up in the morning or after breakfast. Use fluoride toothpaste and a small, soft-bristled brush. Brush all the surfaces of your teeth, especially where they meet the gums, using short, vertical or circular strokes.*

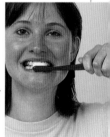

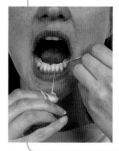

2 *Use dental tape or floss once a day to get rid of plaque between your teeth and at the gum line. Wind a piece around one finger of each hand. Keeping it taut, move it up and down the side of a tooth, going slightly below the gum line. Repeat, using fresh pieces, for every tooth.*

Toothache and sensitive teeth

Toothache can range from a mild ache to a continuous throbbing pain. Tooth decay, usually due to poor dental hygiene, is the most common cause, but pain in the teeth can also be due to gum disease, a cracked tooth, or jaw problems. Teenagers and adults may have pain from wisdom teeth emerging. Your teeth may become sensitive to hot or cold or to brushing if the enamel that protects them becomes worn or cracked, or if your gums recede and expose the inner layers of the teeth.

WARNING

See your dentist immediately or go to an A & E department if you have severe, continuous pain when you bite; fever; foul-smelling breath; and/or a swollen face. You may have a tooth abscess.

 ## See your dentist first

Make an appointment to see your dentist if you are suffering from toothache.

What you can do yourself

Take the following steps to relieve a painful tooth while you are waiting for an appointment with your dentist, or to reduce general sensitivity in your teeth.

- Avoid eating or drinking anything very hot or very cold if this makes the pain worse. Some people, however, find that sucking on an ice cube in the area of the toothache brings relief. Stop if the tooth becomes more painful.

- Rinse your mouth thoroughly with a salt water mouthwash. To make it, mix a teaspoon of salt in a cup of warm water.

 - Try applying oil of cloves to a painful tooth (*see* NATURAL REMEDIES, right).

 - Take a painkiller such as paracetamol or ibuprofen (*see* DRUG REMEDIES, right).

- Use dental tape or floss to remove any food debris trapped between your teeth. Gently clean either side of the painful tooth.

- If you have sensitive teeth, brush your teeth gently using toothpaste formulated for sensitive teeth. After brushing, massage a little toothpaste into your gums and leave it on overnight.

 - Establish a good oral hygiene routine to prevent further tooth decay (*see* PRACTICAL TECHNIQUE, opposite page).

NATURAL REMEDIES

Oil of cloves (*see* p.186) is a traditional remedy from your pharmacist that may help to soothe an aching tooth. Put a few drops of the oil on a piece of cotton wool, place it on the painful tooth, and bite down gently. Be careful to keep the oil off your tongue because it may burn a little.

Clove oil
The oil is distilled from cloves and is antiseptic and anaesthetic, which makes it useful for relieving toothache.

DRUG REMEDIES

Painkillers for toothache include paracetamol (*see* p.187) and ibuprofen (*see* p.184). Try a stronger combined painkiller, such as paracetamol and codeine (*see* p.187), if your tooth is very painful.

- For a child, give paracetamol or ibuprofen to relieve pain and discomfort. They are available in various forms and your pharmacist will advise which is most suitable for your child.

Knocked-out tooth

Teeth are often knocked out during accidents, particularly during contact sports such as rugby. The front teeth are the most vulnerable. If you lose one of your permanent teeth, you may be able to save it by replacing it quickly and getting emergency help. If a tooth is replaced in the socket within about 30 minutes of being knocked out, there is a 90 per cent chance it will be saved, and the chances are still good for up to 2 hours. A broken tooth, however, cannot be saved. Children sometimes lose baby teeth in a fall, but these will be replaced eventually by permanent teeth so there is no need to replace them.

 ### Seek immediate medical advice

If your tooth has been knocked out or loosened by an injury, see your dentist or go to an Accident and Emergency department as soon as possible. If a child loses a baby tooth, it is important to see a dentist to check for possible damage to the mouth or gums.

What you can do yourself

Immediately after the accident, take the following steps to maximize the chances of saving your tooth. Replacing the tooth is the best option, but if you can't do this, you must make sure that the tooth does not dry out while you seek medical help.

- Find the missing tooth and pick it up by the top (the crown), not the root. Do not rub or scrape it to remove dirt or any tissue fragments attached to it. Rinse it gently in a glass of tap water, but don't hold it under running water.

 - Put the tooth back in its socket (*see* PRACTICAL TECHNIQUE, right).

- If you can't replace a permanent tooth in its socket, tuck it under your tongue or inside your cheek. Alternatively, place the tooth in a glass of milk or some of your own saliva.

- If a child has lost a milk tooth and the socket is bleeding, rinse out his or her mouth with water and place a wad of tissue or gauze in the socket. Your child should bite down on it to stop the bleeding.

 ### PRACTICAL TECHNIQUE

Replacing a tooth Whenever possible, you should try to save a permanent tooth by replacing it quickly in the socket. Don't attempt do this, however, if you are concerned that the casualty may swallow or choke on the loose tooth.

1 *Wash your hands thoroughly or put on disposable gloves, if available. Pick up the tooth by the crown and hold it firmly. Check that it is the right way round before pushing it firmly into the socket. Do this even if the socket is bleeding.*

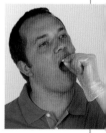

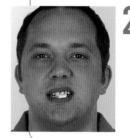

2 *Hold the tooth in place with your fingers, or put a piece of gauze on the tooth and bite down gently on it. Go to a hospital Accident and Emergency department or an emergency dentist for immediate treatment.*

Blocked or runny nose

If you have a runny or blocked nose, you feel stuffed up, may lose your sense of taste and smell, and may only be able to breathe through your mouth. You may cough at night because of mucus dripping down the back of your throat. If your "bunged up" nose is due to a cold or sinus infection, you may also have a thick yellowish-green discharge from your nose. A blocked or runny nose can also be caused by allergies to substances such as pollen, house dust mites, pet dander (flakes of skin), and mould. Symptoms can occur at any time or be seasonal, as with hay fever.

 See also Common cold, p.78; Sinusitis, p.79; Hay fever, p.80; Coughing, p.102.

What you can do yourself

Try the following home treatments to help relieve your blocked or runny nose.

 ● Drink at least 8 glasses a day of clear fluids such as water, fruit juice, herbal teas, and clear soups. Hot drinks will help to loosen mucus if your nose is blocked. Using saline nose drops has a similar effect (*see* DRUG REMEDIES, right).

● Try a steam inhalation, or run hot water into the bath or shower and inhale the steam (*see* PRACTICAL TECHNIQUE: STEAM INHALATION, p.79).

 ● Remedies containing aromatic oils may help to relieve a stuffy nose (*see* NATURAL REMEDIES, right).

 ● If you have a blocked nose due to a cold, try a decongestant nasal spray (*see* DRUG REMEDIES, right).

● If your nose is sore from blowing it, apply some petroleum jelly around your nostrils to protect them.

 ● To treat a blocked or runny nose caused by an allergy, use a steroid nasal spray and/or an oral antihistamine (*see* DRUG REMEDIES, right).

● Avoid smoke and dust; they can irritate the lining of your nose and worsen symptoms.

Seek medical advice

Arrange to see your doctor if:

● Symptoms have not begun to clear up using the measures described here
● You develop new symptoms
● You are using medications continually to relieve your blocked or runny nose

NATURAL REMEDIES

Aromatic oils (*see* p.178) such as menthol, eucalyptus, or camphor, are traditional treatments for a blocked nose. Try sucking lozenges containing menthol, or putting a few drops of an aromatic oil on a tissue and inhaling it. Use a menthol chest rub at night if you are having difficulty sleeping.

DRUG REMEDIES

Saline nose drops (*see* p.188) can be bought from your pharmacist, or you can make your own by dissolving half a teaspoon of salt in 250 ml (half a pint) of lukewarm water. Apply them using a dropper, 2–4 times a day.

Decongestants (*see* p.181), available as nasal sprays or drops, quickly relieve a blocked nose by reducing swelling and congestion in the tissues lining the nose. They also lessen mucus production. They should not, however, be used for more than 7 days, otherwise they may make you feel more blocked up when you stop using them.

Steroid nasal sprays (*see* p.188) containing a corticosteroid drug are particularly effective for nasal symptoms such as a blocked nose. They can take several days to reach their full effect, so, if possible, start using them at least 2–3 days before exposure to allergic triggers.

Antihistamines (*see* p.178), in the form of tablets or liquids, usually work within 1 hour. You can use them to relieve a runny nose due to allergy, but they are not so effective for a blocked nose. They can be taken regularly or only as needed – for example, if you are visiting a house with pets.

Common cold

Colds are common infections of the nose and throat that can be caused by more than 200 different, highly contagious viruses. You are likely to pick up at least one or two colds a year, usually from the coughs and sneezes of infected people. Children are even more susceptible because they have not built up immunity to cold viruses. Typical symptoms are a blocked or runny nose, sneezing, reduced sense of taste and smell, sore throat, a dry cough, headache, and mild fever. Colds can be more serious in babies and elderly people.

 See also Blocked or runny nose, p.77; Sore throat, p.81; Headache, p.85.

What you can do yourself

Most people recover from a cold within a week, but there are things you can do to make yourself feel better in the meantime.

- Drink at least 8 glasses of warm liquids a day such as fruit teas and clear soups. Avoid tea and coffee. To relieve a sore throat, make a warm honey and lemon drink (*see* NATURAL REMEDIES, p.30).

- Take a painkiller or a cold remedy to relieve discomfort (*see* DRUG REMEDIES, right).

- Try a steam inhalation to clear a stuffy nose (*see* PRACTICAL TECHNIQUE, opposite page). You can also use saline nose drops (*see* DRUG REMEDIES, opposite page) or a decongestant (*see* DRUG REMEDIES, right).

- Use paper tissues rather than handkerchiefs to blow your nose. If your nose is sore, try tissues with soothing ingredients such as aloe vera.

- Antihistamines may help to relieve a runny nose and reduce sneezing (*see* DRUG REMEDIES, right).

- You may be able to speed your recovery by taking zinc, and relieve the worst symptoms of a cold with echinacea (*see* NATURAL REMEDIES, right).

- Do not smoke, and avoid smoky environments.

Seek medical advice

Arrange to see your doctor if:

- Your cold persists for more than 10 days
- You develop a severe sore throat or high fever, or cough up yellow or green mucus
- You have earache or face pain and/or a greenish-yellow nasal discharge

DRUG REMEDIES

Painkillers Paracetamol (*see* p.187), aspirin (*see* p.179), or ibuprofen (see p.184) can help to relieve headache, fever, and sore throat.

CAUTION: Don't give aspirin to children under 16, except on the advice of your doctor.

Cold and flu remedies (*see* p.179) contain painkillers, decongestants, and antihistamines to relieve a range of symptoms. Don't use them with other painkillers because of the risk of overdose.

Decongestants (*see* p.181) in the form of nasal sprays or drops containing xylometazoline or oxymetazoline can help to clear a blocked-up nose.

Antihistamines (*see* p.178) can help clear up a runny nose and sneezing, although they tend to dry out the nasal passages.

NATURAL REMEDIES

Zinc lozenges, taken early on in a cold, may help to shorten the illness. Occasionally, they cause a bad taste in the mouth and mild nausea.

Echinacea (*see* p.181), taken as a tincture or capsules, can help to reduce cold symptoms and speed recovery.

Using echinacea
The herb is most effective when taken at the start of a cold.

Sinusitis

Sinusitis is an inflammation of the membranes lining the sinuses, which are air-filled pockets located behind the nose, cheeks, and forehead. It causes pain and tenderness around your eyes and cheeks; a stuffy and/or runny nose; and, sometimes, aching in your upper teeth and jaw. You may also have a foul taste in your mouth and feel feverish. Sinusitis is usually a complication of an infection such as a cold or flu. People who swim or dive regularly may be more susceptible than is usual to the problem.

> **WARNING**
>
> Seek immediate medical help if you also develop severe headaches, vomiting, and fever.

See your doctor first

Make an appointment to see your doctor if you think you may have sinusitis, to confirm the diagnosis and get advice on treatment.

What you can do yourself

You can do several things to relieve the "bunged-up" feeling of sinusitis and speed your recovery.

● Put a warm, moist face cloth over your nose to relieve pain, or use steam inhalation up to 3–4 times a day to reduce congestion (see PRACTICAL TECHNIQUE, right).

● If you are in pain or have a fever, take a painkiller (see DRUG REMEDIES, right).

● Drink at least 8 glasses of warm fluids a day.

● Decongestants may help to clear your nose. Alternatively, try using saline nose drops to loosen mucus. (see DRUG REMEDIES, right.)

● Blow your nose gently.

● Get plenty of rest. Sleep with your head raised. Sleeping on your side may make breathing easier.

● Try to avoid spending time in cold, polluted, or smoky atmospheres.

Seek further medical advice

Arrange to see your doctor if your sinusitis has not begun to clear up after a few days.

PRACTICAL TECHNIQUE

Steam inhalation This helps loosen mucus in the nose, throat, and sinuses. Children should only use steam inhalations if supervised by an adult.

● Fill a bowl one-third full with hot, but not boiling, water. You can add eucalyptus oil, pine oil, or menthol (see AROMATIC OILS, p.178) to make it smell pleasant.
● Lean forwards, cover your head and the bowl with a towel, and gently inhale the steam. If your nose is blocked, breathe through your mouth until your nose clears.

Inhaling steam
Breathe in and out through your nose for several minutes.

DRUG REMEDIES

Painkillers, such as paracetamol (see p.187) and ibuprofen (see p.184), will help to relieve pain around the eyes and cheeks and bring down a fever. If the pain is severe, try a painkiller that combines paracetamol and codeine (see p.187).

Decongestants (see p.181) help to reduce swelling inside the nose and sinuses.

Saline nose drops (see p.188) can be used up to 6 times a day to help loosen mucus in the nasal passages.

Hay fever

Hay fever is caused by an allergy to pollen or mould. When pollen grains or mould spores get into your eyes, nose, or airways, they cause symptoms such as sneezing; a runny or blocked nose; itching in your eyes, nose, and the roof of your mouth; watery, red eyes; and a cough. You may also develop wheezing. Symptoms can develop at any time from early spring to early autumn, depending on which pollens or moulds trigger the allergy. Hay fever tends to run in families that have a high incidence of allergic conditions such as asthma and eczema, but many people seem to grow out of the problem as they get older.

 See also Conjunctivitis, p.58; Blocked or runny nose, p.77; Wheezing, p.103.

What you can do yourself

Most people are able to control their symptoms using over-the-counter remedies. Try the following to see what works best for you.

 ● Take an antihistamine to relieve most hay fever symptoms (*see* DRUG REMEDIES, right).

 A steroid nasal spray is particularly effective in helping to prevent or relieve sneezing, watering, itching, and stuffiness in your nose (*see* DRUG REMEDIES, right). You can use the spray either alone or with an antihistamine.

 ● Sodium cromoglicate nasal spray (*see* DRUG REMEDIES, right) can be used as an alternative to a steroid nasal spray for mild symptoms.

 ● For itchy eyes, use sodium cromoglicate or antihistamine eye drops (*see* DRUG REMEDIES, right).

 ● Decongestant drugs can be used in the short term to clear a blocked nose (*see* DRUG REMEDIES, right). They can also be used to help clear your nose when starting a course of a steroid nasal spray.

 ● Avoid substances that can further irritate your nose and eyes, such as tobacco smoke or dust, perfumes, or strong-smelling chemicals.

● When the pollen count is high (usually on hot, dry, windy days at mid-morning and early evening), stay indoors as much as possible, keeping windows and doors closed. In a car, keep windows and air vents closed. Some newer cars have pollen filters.

● Dry clothes inside if possible. If you do dry washing outside, bring it in before the evening.

● Have a shower and wash your hair before bed to remove pollen that has built up during the day.

DRUG REMEDIES

Antihistamine tablets (*see* p.178) are a convenient treatment that can be used on a one-off basis or regularly, and with nose sprays or eye drops (if these treatments don't ease symptoms by themselves). They quickly relieve most hay fever symptoms, including sneezing, although they are not as effective as steroids for a blocked nose.

Steroid nasal sprays (*see* p.188) relieve nasal symptoms more effectively than antihistamines. They can take several days to reach their full effect, so try to start the treatment before the hay fever season begins, and use the spray daily.

Sodium cromoglicate nasal spray (*see* p.188) can be used as an alternative to a steroid nasal spray, although it is not generally as effective. It also needs to be used continuously.

Eye drops containing sodium cromoglicate (*see* p.188) or antihistamine (*see* p.178) can prevent or relieve symptoms. Sodium cromoglicate eye drops can take a few days to have a noticeable effect, and they must be used continuously.

Decongestants (*see* p.181), available as nasal sprays or drops, act quickly. They are good for occasional use. Do not use them for more than 7 days, however, or they may make you feel more blocked up when you stop.

 ### Seek medical advice

Arrange to see your doctor if:

● There is no improvement after you have been using home treatments for 2–3 weeks

Sore throat

Sore throats are very common. As well as a painful throat, you may have difficulty swallowing, a mild cough, hoarse voice, fever, headache, and enlarged glands in the front of your neck. Normally, the soreness gets worse over a period of 2–3 days, then begins to clear up. A sore throat is usually caused by a viral infection, and often develops with a cold or flu. It may also be a symptom of glandular fever. Another possible cause is tonsillitis – an infection of the tonsils at the back of the throat. If you have tonsillitis, you are likely to feel even more feverish and generally unwell. Your tonsils will be enlarged and may have pus on them, and your throat will feel uncomfortable when you try to eat or drink.

What you can do yourself

Use these home treatments to make your throat feel more comfortable while you get better.

● Drink at least 8 glasses of fluids a day, even if this feels painful, because your throat will feel worse if it is dry and/or if you become dehydrated. Drinks such as warm honey and lemon are particularly soothing (*see* NATURAL REMEDIES, p.30). Avoid undiluted citrus juices because they are acidic and may irritate your throat.

 ● Try a throat treatment: suck a lozenge or use a spray containing a local anaesthetic to numb your throat (*see* DRUG REMEDIES, right).

● Have bland, soft foods, such as rice pudding and yoghurt, while your throat is sore. Ice cream is cooling and soothing. It will also help to encourage a child with a sore throat to eat.

 ● Take a painkiller or try a pain-relieving gargle (*see* DRUG REMEDIES, right).

● You can also gargle with a salt solution. Dissolve half a teaspoon of salt in a glass of warm water, gargle for 30 seconds, then spit it out.

● Don't use mouthwashes containing alcohol because they will dry your mouth and tongue.

● Rest your voice. Avoid talking too much or straining your voice.

● Keep your rooms humidified to keep your throat moist. Put a bowl of water in a room, hang a wet towel close to a radiator, or use a humidifier.

● Avoid spending time in smoky or polluted environments because this will make your symptoms worse. If you smoke, try to stop or at least cut down while you have a sore throat.

DRUG REMEDIES

Mouth and throat treatments (*see* p.186) containing anaesthetics will numb a sore throat temporarily and make it easier for you to drink and eat. You can also use benzydamine, an anti-inflammatory painkiller available as a rinse, spray, or gargle. Gargles may not be suitable for children.

Painkillers Take paracetamol (*see* p.187) or ibuprofen (*see* p.184). Give a child paracetamol liquid, soluble tablets, or melt-in-the-mouth tablets, or ibuprofen liquid. Adults can also gargle with 1 or 2 soluble aspirin (*see* p.179) dissolved in water; repeat 3–4 times a day as necessary.

CAUTION: Don't give aspirin to children under 16 unless on a doctor's advice.

Pain relief
Tilt your head back and gargle with the solution or rinse for 1–2 minutes before spitting it out.

 ### Seek medical advice

Arrange to see your doctor if:

● A sore throat becomes more severe or has not got better after 5 days
● You are finding it very difficult to swallow
● You develop other symptoms, such as joint pains or swellings in your armpits or groin

Hoarseness and loss of voice

When your voice sounds scratchy or husky and you have difficulty making yourself heard, the cause is usually inflammation of the voice box (laryngitis) due to an infection such as a cold. Your throat may be sore as well or feel as if there is a lump in it. You can also suddenly lose your voice as a result of overuse – for example, after shouting at a football match. When hoarseness develops gradually, it is usually because of prolonged overuse of the voice, smoking, or reflux of stomach acid (heartburn) irritating the voice box. In rare cases, a hoarse voice is a symptom of cancer of the larynx.

 See also Sore throat, p.81; Heartburn, p.107.

What you can do yourself

Hoarseness and loss of voice are usually temporary, lasting for no more than a week. The following measures will help you recover your voice.

● Rest your voice as much as possible. Don't talk or whisper. Whispering can strain your vocal cords even more than normal speech.

● Drink plenty of warm fluids to soothe your throat and 6–8 glasses of water a day to keep it lubricated. Don't drink caffeinated drinks or alcohol.

● Eat soft foods that can be swallowed easily.

● Avoid dry or smoky environments, which can dry the throat and aggravate hoarseness.

 ● If your throat feels sore, take a painkiller (*see* DRUG REMEDIES, right).

● Try a steam inhalation to soothe inflammation and loosen secretions (*see* PRACTICAL TECHNIQUE: STEAM INHALATION, p.79).

● Don't gargle – it does not help, and the alcohol in some gargles may cause more irritation. Cough medicines won't relieve hoarseness, either.

Seek medical advice

Arrange to see your doctor promptly if:

● Your throat is still hoarse after 2 weeks
● You are also having difficulty breathing or swallowing

DRUG REMEDIES

Painkillers, such as paracetamol (*see* p.187), will help to relieve the discomfort if your throat is painful as well as hoarse.

PREVENTION

Protecting your throat If you are prone to hoarseness and losing your voice, try using the following measures to help prevent recurrences.

● Drink 6–8 glasses of water a day. Keep a bottle of water on your desk at work, and take frequent sips.
● If your work involves speaking to a group or class, try to avoid raising or straining your voice. Organize smaller groups and sit closer together. If you need to address a large audience, ask for a microphone.
● Shouting or screaming puts unnecessary strain on your voice, so try to control anger or anxiety if it makes you prone to doing this.
● Stop smoking and avoid spending long periods in smoky atmospheres.
● Try not to cough or clear your throat forcibly.
● Try to breathe through your nose. Breathing through your mouth dries the lining of your throat and introduces cold, unfiltered air into the lungs, which contributes to hoarseness.
● Use a humidifier in your home, or place bowls of water beside a radiator, to keep the air moist.

Nosebleed

Nosebleeds are common in children, but some adults have them occasionally, too. Common causes include nose-picking and forceful nose-blowing, but nosebleeds often occur for no obvious reason. Your nose is more likely to bleed if its delicate lining is irritated because of a cold or an allergy, or if it becomes dry and cracked due to a dry atmosphere. Although most nosebleeds are little more than a temporary nuisance, bleeding is sometimes a symptom of an underlying illness.

WARNING

Seek immediate medical help if:
- Bleeding is very severe
- You have hit your head or neck
- You are vomiting swallowed blood
- You are taking aspirin or any blood-thinning medication

What you can do yourself

Nosebleeds may look alarming but can usually be stopped fairly easily and prevented from restarting. In older people, a nosebleed can be more difficult to control. Try the following measures.

Controlling a nosebleed
- Stay calm. If you are helping someone else with a nosebleed, be reassuring.

- Take steps to stop the bleeding (see PRACTICAL TECHNIQUE, right).

- Don't push tissue or cotton wool into your nostrils to try to stop the bleeding.

Once bleeding has stopped
- Try not to blow your nose for 24 hours afterwards. Make sure that you don't pick your nose.

- If you feel the need to sneeze, do so with your mouth open.

- Avoid drinking hot liquids or alcohol, or smoking.

- Sleep with your head raised on 2 or 3 pillows.

- Avoid vigorous exercise for 24 hours after a nosebleed has occurred.

- In dry, centrally heated rooms, use a humidifier or place a bowl of water close to a radiator.

- If you are prone to nosebleeds because your nose tends to be dry and crusted inside, rub petroleum jelly inside your nostrils a few times a day to soften and protect the delicate membrane that lines the nose. Alternatively, use saline nose drops to keep the nasal membrane moist (see DRUG REMEDIES, right).

PRACTICAL TECHNIQUE

Stopping a nosebleed These steps should stop a nosebleed within 5–10 minutes.
- Lean forwards slightly. If you are feeling faint, sit down and lean forwards.
- Firmly pinch the soft part of your nose for 5–10 minutes. Breathe through your mouth.
- If bleeding persists after 10 minutes, pinch for another 5–10 minutes. If this does not work, seek immediate medical help.

Pinching your nose
Pinch the soft part just below the bridge.

DRUG REMEDIES

Saline nose drops (see p.188) are available from your pharmacist and are safe to use on children. If the lining of your nose is dry, use them several times a day.

 Seek medical advice

Arrange to see your doctor if:
- You are getting recurrent nosebleeds
- You are feeling generally unwell
- You are bruising easily

Snoring

Snoring is the sound of the soft palate (the back of the roof of the mouth) vibrating when it relaxes during sleep. Although it does no harm in itself, it can disturb the snorer and anyone who shares the same bed or room. Snoring can be provoked by conditions that cause swelling in the nasal and throat passages, such as hay fever, colds, and throat or sinus infections, as well as combinations of lifestyle factors such as drinking alcohol, being overweight, and smoking. More men than women snore, and the tendency to do so increases from middle age onwards. In children, it is often due to enlarged tonsils and adenoids.

 ### See your doctor first

Make an appointment to see your doctor if you or your partner notice the following symptom in addition to snoring:

● You have pauses in breathing of 10 seconds or more during sleep. (You may wake suddenly as you take a deep breath to compensate.)

What you can do yourself

As well as being embarrassing, snoring can be disruptive to relationships. Try some of the following measures to get a better night's sleep.

● You are more likely to snore when sleeping on your back. Train yourself to sleep on your side by tucking a pillow into your back or sewing a tennis ball into the back of your nightclothes.

● Lose any excess weight; this will reduce fat deposits around the back of your mouth and nose.

● Reduce your alcohol intake and avoid drinking any alcohol in the 4–5 hours before you go to bed.

● Give up smoking, as tobacco smoke irritates the linings of the nose and throat.

● Don't use sleeping tablets or sedative antihistamines because they relax the soft palate.

● Try self-help measures to relieve any nasal congestion (see BLOCKED OR RUNNY NOSE, p.77).

 ● It may help to use a plaster strip that keeps the nasal passages open (see PRACTICAL TECHNIQUE, right).

● If your partner's snoring is making it impossible for you to sleep, try gently nudging or calling to your partner so that he or she changes position but does not wake up.

 PRACTICAL TECHNIQUE

Using a nasal strip One remedy for snoring uses an adhesive strip attached to the nose to make breathing easier. Stick the strip across the soft part of your nose before you go to bed. The adhesive pad has bands of plastic embedded in it that tighten and lift the sides of the nose, helping to maintain airflow while you sleep.

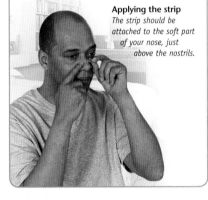

Applying the strip
The strip should be attached to the soft part of your nose, just above the nostrils.

 ### Seek further medical advice

Arrange to see your doctor if:

● The snoring is not helped by the measures on this page and is disrupting your sleep and/or your partner's sleep
● You feel tired and irritable during the day

HEAD, BACK, AND LIMB PROBLEMS

Headache

The most common type of headache is a tension headache. You may feel pressure around your head and behind your eyes and have a stiff neck and shoulder muscles. Tension headaches usually last for a few hours and are commonly due to stress, tiredness, or poor posture, which may cause tension in the neck and scalp. Other triggers include certain foods, poor eyesight, hunger or dehydration, and hormonal changes in the menstrual cycle. Headaches also occur with illnesses such as flu and can be a symptom of meningitis.

 WARNING

Seek urgent medical attention if the pain is sudden and incapacitating, follows head injury, or occurs with:
● Drowsiness and blurred vision
● Stiff neck; sensitivity to light; fever; vomiting; possibly a rash (*see* p.150)
● Limb weakness

 See also Migraine, p.86.

What you can do yourself

Use the following measures at the first sign of a headache to stop it from becoming worse.

 ● Take a painkiller (*see* DRUG REMEDIES, right). It is best to start taking it as soon as the headache begins, before the pain becomes intense.

● Have a hot bath or shower to help your neck and shoulder muscles relax.

● Try using heat to soothe the pain: fill a hot-water bottle, wrap it in a towel, and rest your head on it.

● Ask a partner or friend to massage the muscles at the back of your neck, using his or her fingertips in a gentle circular motion.

● Rest in a quiet room, in darkness or with dimmed lights. Make sure you get enough sleep at night.

● If headaches are linked to stress, try aerobic exercise (such as brisk walking), yoga, or practise deep breathing and muscle relaxation exercises (*see* PRACTICAL TECHNIQUES, pp.20–21).

● Have your eyesight checked.

● If you work at a desk or computer workstation, get up and walk around regularly to reduce tension in your neck and shoulders.

● Avoid drinking alcohol and caffeine in excess, and smoking, all of which can lead to headaches.

 DRUG REMEDIES

Painkillers Take ibuprofen (*see* p.184) or paracetamol (*see* p.187) for a headache, but don't use painkillers for more than a few days at a time. If you take them regularly your body will become accustomed to them and you may have continuing headaches as each dose of medication wears off.

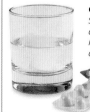

Choosing painkillers
Soluble painkillers and liquid capsules are absorbed fast. Melt-in-the-mouth tablets dissolve on the tongue.

 Seek medical advice

Arrange to see your doctor if:

● The headache has not cleared up within a day or two or is becoming more severe
● You feel that your headache is not a simple tension headache
● You have recurrent headaches or need to use painkillers regularly

Migraine

A migraine is an intense, throbbing headache, usually on one side of your head and often behind one eye or temple. You may feel nauseous or vomit, and be particularly sensitive to bright light and loud noises. A migraine can last for anything from a few hours to 3 days and may be so debilitating that it prevents normal activities. Shortly before an attack, some people have warning symptoms (known as aura), such as visual disturbances and an altered sense of taste and smell. Factors that can trigger migraines in susceptible people include stress; changes in sleep routine; certain foods and drinks; and, in women, fluctuating hormone levels.

 ## See your doctor first

Make an appointment to see your doctor to confirm that your symptoms are due to migraine.

What you can do yourself

Use the following treatments and self-help measures as soon as an attack begins.

- Take a painkiller at the first sign of an attack. If you feel sick or are vomiting, take a migraine remedy (*see* DRUG REMEDIES, right).

- If possible, lie down in a dark, quiet room with pillows to support your head. Try to sleep.

- Sip water throughout the day, especially if you have been vomiting.

- Wear sunglasses if you are out in bright daylight.

 ### PREVENTION

Reducing attacks To reduce the frequency and severity of migraine attacks, try these measures.

- Keep a diary for a few weeks, noting when you have migraines and any possible contributory factors. Foods such as red wine, chocolate, and cheese are common triggers. Taking too much caffeine or cutting back suddenly on your regular intake can cause migraine.
- If stress is a factor, try to reduce it (*see* pp.20–21).
- Eat regularly and drink 6–8 glasses of water a day.
- Keep to a regular sleep pattern. Too little or too much sleep can trigger a migraine.
- Taking the herb feverfew may help to prevent migraine attacks (*see* NATURAL REMEDIES, right).

DRUG REMEDIES

Painkillers, such as paracetamol (*see* p.187), aspirin (*see* p.179), or ibuprofen (*see* p.184), should be taken as soon as symptoms or aura begin to develop. Soluble tablets may work more quickly. If these are not effective, try paracetamol and codeine (*see* p.187). **CAUTION:** Don't give aspirin to anyone under 16 years.

Migraine remedies (*see* p.185) include painkillers and an anti-nausea drug in one tablet. Alternatively, take prochlorperazine tablets, which are dissolved on the gum to relieve nausea and vomiting. Take these with your usual painkiller.

NATURAL REMEDIES

Feverfew (*see* p.182) is a garden herb that is available as supplements. Some people find that it reduces the frequency of migraine attacks.

Feverfew capsules
Try taking the capsules for a few weeks to see if they help.

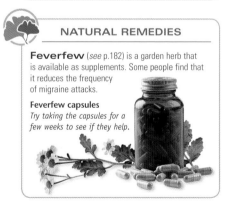

 ## Seek further medical advice

Arrange to see your doctor if:

- Your migraines are not getting better with self-help or prescribed treatments
- You are having frequent or severe attacks

Sore or stiff neck

A painful or stiff neck is usually due to a muscle strain or spasm, caused by poor posture or a minor injury. You may suffer from a stiff neck and shoulders if you sit hunched over a computer for long periods, or you may wake with a stiff neck if you sleep awkwardly. Pain may also be felt in your head, shoulders, arms, or upper back and may be worse when you turn your head or look up or down. Pain and stiffness can also be due to a "whiplash injury", arthritis in the spine, or an underlying illness or injury.

> ### WARNING
>
> Seek immediate medical help if:
>
> • You have a sore or stiff neck with any or all of the following symptoms: fever, vomiting, headache, dislike of bright light, and a rash (see p.150)

See your doctor first

Make an appointment to see your doctor if:

• You have a sore or stiff neck after an injury
• You have tingling, numbness, or weakness in an arm or hand, or weight loss or fever

What you can do yourself

A stiff and sore neck due to muscle strain or poor posture should begin to ease within 2–3 days using these home treatments.

• Continue with normal activities as far as the pain allows. If the pain is bad, however, you may need to rest your neck for the first day or two.

• A padded collar may help to support your neck. You can make a collar by rolling up a hand towel and putting it into one leg of a pair of tights, then gently securing it around your neck. Only wear a collar for a short period, and don't wear it at night.

 • Start gentle neck exercises as soon as you are able to do so (see PRACTICAL TECHNIQUE, right).

 • Take a painkiller or try an ibuprofen gel or cream (see DRUG REMEDIES, right).

• To relieve muscle spasm, stand under a warm shower, or place a covered hot-water bottle or a heating pad on the back of your neck, for 15 minutes every few hours.

• Use a supportive pillow in bed. Alternatively, make a neck-support pillow by tying a scarf or bandage around the middle of a pillow to form a butterfly shape. Rest your head on the narrow part.

PRACTICAL TECHNIQUE

Neck exercise The following exercise will help to loosen up a stiff neck.

• Stand straight, or sit on the edge of a chair looking straight ahead. Drop your head to one side, towards your shoulder. Keep your shoulder down.
• Hold for a few seconds, then raise your head again. Repeat on the other side.
• Repeat the exercise 5 times on each side, about 3 times a day. Exercise to the point of discomfort, but don't try to exercise through pain.
• Gradually increase the range of movement. Stop at once, however, if the pain gets worse or if it begins to move into your arm or hand.

DRUG REMEDIES

Painkillers will help relieve the discomfort of a stiff or sore neck and help you to keep your neck mobile. Take paracetamol (see p.187), or ibuprofen (see p.184), which may be more effective.

Ibuprofen gels and creams (see p.184) have an anti-inflammatory effect and may reduce pain when rubbed into the neck area.

Seek further medical advice

Arrange to see your doctor if:

• The soreness or stiffness is getting worse
• The problem has not eased after 2 days

Lower back pain

Most sudden back pain is due to a sprain or a small tear in a muscle or ligament. You may have a niggling ache in your lower back or a sharp, localized pain and stiffness due to muscle spasm in the area. Sciatica is pain that travels through one buttock to the leg and foot, sometimes with numbness, tingling, and weakness in the leg. It is caused by trapping or irritation of the sciatic nerve, often due to a "slipped disc" between the bones of the spine. The usual causes of back pain and sciatica include lifting awkwardly or sudden twisting, but factors such as poor posture, pregnancy, and being inactive or unfit may make the back more vulnerable.

> **WARNING**
>
> Seek immediate medical help if:
> - You have difficulty controlling your bowels or bladder; tingling and/or numbness in the anal or genital area; or muscle weakness
> - Back pain follows an injury

 ## See your doctor first

Make an appointment to see your doctor if:

- You have symptoms of sciatica
- Back pain has been developing slowly and is gradually getting worse
- You are losing weight or have a fever

What you can do yourself

An episode of back pain usually gets better within a few weeks. Take these steps to ease pain, staying as active as possible rather than resting in bed.

- If the pain is tolerable, try to continue normal activities as much as possible. Gradually increase what you do each day, but don't overdo things. Stop any activity that makes the pain worse.

- If the pain is so severe that you cannot move, rest in bed for a day or two. As soon as you feel able to do so, get out of bed and start moving, even if it causes some discomfort.

- Your mattress needs to be firm, but not too hard. If you have an old, sagging mattress that does not support your back, put a board under it. You will probably find that lying on your side is more comfortable than lying on your back.

 - While your back is painful, try to move in ways that are less likely to bring on or worsen the pain (*see* PRACTICAL TECHNIQUE, right).

 - Take painkillers to relieve pain and stiffness (*see* DRUG REMEDIES, opposite page).

PRACTICAL TECHNIQUE

Moving without pain Getting out of bed awkwardly can cause sudden, painful twinges when you have back pain. This sequence of movements will get you on your feet with the minimum strain on your spine, so continue to use them even when your back is no longer painful.

1 *Lying flat on your back, bring your knees up to hip level and roll yourself slowly on to your side, facing the edge of the bed.*

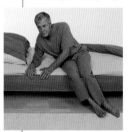

2 *Swing your legs to the edge of the bed and lower your feet to the floor. Use your arms to push yourself into a sitting position.*

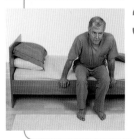

3 *Using your arms and your leg muscles to push yourself up, slowly rise to a standing position. Reverse the procedure when you get back into bed.*

What you can do yourself *continued...*

- Rub ibuprofen gel or cream into the area to ease pain and inflammation (*see* DRUG REMEDIES, right).

- Rubbing the sore area with a counter-irritant cream or gel may help to soothe the pain for a short while (*see* DRUG REMEDIES, right).

- Holding a wrapped hot-water bottle or heating pad against your back may help to relieve pain, particularly if there is muscle spasm. You can also direct warm water on to the small of your back when in the shower.

Seek further medical advice

Arrange to see your doctor if:

- The back pain is getting worse or is not easing within 48 hours
- You develop any of the symptoms listed in the Warning box

PREVENTION

Avoiding back pain If you are prone to back pain, you may be able to prevent further episodes by taking particular care of your back.

- Wear comfortable shoes with a low heel.
- If you are overweight, lose weight – it will help to take pressure off your back.
- Walking, swimming, or a course of Pilates or yoga exercises will help to strengthen your back muscles. Your doctor or physiotherapist can also recommend back-strengthening exercises.
- Try to improve your posture when you walk, stand, and sit, both while you have back pain and afterwards (*see* PRACTICAL TECHNIQUE, right). You should also practise safe ways of lifting and moving heavy objects to reduce the risk of straining your back (*see* PREVENTION: LIFTING HEAVY OBJECTS, p.112).

DRUG REMEDIES

Painkillers include paracetamol (*see* p.187) and ibuprofen (*see* p.184). Ibuprofen also has an anti-inflammatory effect, which will reduce stiffness, making it easier for you to try some gentle movement. If pain persists, try a stronger painkiller containing paracetamol and codeine (*see* p.187).

Ibuprofen gel, cream, or spray (*see* p.184) has an anti-inflammatory effect and reduces pain when you apply it directly to the affected area.

Counter-irritants (*see* p.180), available as creams, gels, or sprays, produce a tingling sensation in the skin that soothes pain temporarily. Some warm the area; others have a cooling effect.

PRACTICAL TECHNIQUES

Standing and walking When you are standing or walking, pull your shoulders slightly back and down, holding your trunk straight. Try to balance your weight evenly over both feet.

Driving Angle the driver's seat backwards very slightly and position it so you can reach the hand and foot controls easily. While you are driving, check from time to time that your arms are relaxed and your shoulders are not hunched.

Sitting Sit with your back straight, your bottom pushed into the back of a chair, and your feet flat on the floor. Choose a chair that is the right height to allow you to do this, with an upright back that supports the small of your back. The seat should support the full length of your thighs but should not put too much pressure on the backs of your thighs. When using a computer, the top of the screen should be at eye level.

Good posture
Sit well back in the chair, with your back straight and your lower back supported by the backrest. Keep both feet flat on the floor.

Shoulder pain

Shoulder pain can be continuous or it may occur only when you make certain movements, such as circling your arm. The pain may also radiate down one arm. The usual cause is inflammation of the muscles and tendons that surround the shoulder joint. This may develop if you strain your shoulder, for example during sport or other strenuous activities. Gradual wear and tear on the joint from osteoarthritis can also cause shoulder pain.

> **WARNING**
>
> Seek immediate medical help if shoulder pain is associated with:
> - Pain or heaviness in your chest
> - Sweating
> - Breathlessness

 ## See your doctor first

Make an appointment to see your doctor if you have shoulder pain after a fall or injury.

What you can do yourself

There are several things you can do to reduce pain and stiffness and get your shoulder moving normally.

- Take a painkiller, or rub in a preparation containing ibuprofen (*see* DRUG REMEDIES, right).

- Apply an ice pack (such as a bag of frozen peas or crushed ice, wrapped in a wet towel). Hold for 10 minutes. Reapply 2–3 times a day for the first 2 days.

- Massaging a counter-irritant cream or gel into the sore area may help to soothe the pain for a short while (*see* DRUG REMEDIES, right).

- Rest the shoulder for a few days, but try to keep it mobile by gently shrugging from time to time. If you don't, it may get persistently stiff and painful ("frozen shoulder"). As the pain eases, start exercising your shoulder (*see* PRACTICAL TECHNIQUE, right).

- At night, lie on the pain-free side and cuddle a cushion with the other arm for support. If you lie on your back, support your arm with a pillow.

- Make sure you keep your armpit on the affected side clean and dry to avoid soreness.

Seek further medical advice

Arrange to see your doctor if:

- Your shoulder is becoming more painful
- It is not getting better after 2–3 days

 ### DRUG REMEDIES

Painkillers Take paracetamol (*see* p.187) or ibuprofen (*see* p.184) to relieve pain. Ibuprofen has an anti-inflammatory effect, which will help reduce swelling and stiffness. Ibuprofen gel, cream, or spray has similar painkilling and anti-inflammatory effects and is applied directly to the affected area.

Counter-irritants (*see* p.180) are creams and gels that produce a tingling sensation in the skin, which soothes pain temporarily.

PRACTICAL TECHNIQUE

Shoulder exercises Do these exercises twice a day to improve flexibility. You may find it helpful to do them under a warm shower. Gradually increase the range of movement as the pain lessens.

1 *Put your arms out to the side and lift them, stopping as soon as it becomes uncomfortable. Slowly drop them to your sides. Repeat 5 times.*

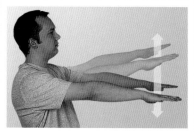

2 *Put your arms out to the front and lift them until you start to feel discomfort. Slowly drop them to your sides. Repeat 5 times.*

Tennis or golfer's elbow

Also called tendinitis, tennis or golfer's elbow is inflammation of the tendons where they attach to the bone at the elbow. The main symptom is pain in the forearm that becomes worse when you try to pick up objects, shake hands, or use any action that puts strain on the affected tendon. Overuse of your wrist and forearm while playing sports is the usual cause, although inflammation can also occur when you use a screwdriver or similar tool too vigorously. Tennis elbow affects the tendon on the outer side of your elbow, and golfer's elbow involves the tendon on the inner side.

 ## See your doctor first

Make an appointment to see your doctor if:

- You develop pain in your elbow after an injury
- Your elbow is swollen and feels hot

What you can do yourself

There are several ways to reduce elbow pain. It's important to start treatment as soon as possible.

- Rest your arm and hand whenever you can, and reduce activities that put strain on the tendon.

- Apply an ice pack (such as a bag of frozen peas or crushed ice, wrapped in a wet towel) to the painful area. Hold in place for about 10 minutes. Reapply 2–3 times a day for the first 2 days.

- Try wearing an elbow strap, available from your pharmacist, to help ease the pain of tendinitis.

 - Take a painkiller, or rub in a preparation containing ibuprofen (*see* DRUG REMEDIES, right).

- Massaging a counter-irritant into the sore area may help to soothe pain (*see* DRUG REMEDIES, right).

- When you are ready to resume playing sports, practise elbow-stretching exercises before you play (*see* PRACTICAL TECHNIQUE, right). Ask your doctor or physiotherapist for advice on other exercises to strengthen your elbow joint.

 ## Seek further medical advice

Arrange to see your doctor if:

- The pain does not start to subside after 1–2 weeks of the treatment described above

 ### DRUG REMEDIES

Painkillers Take paracetamol (*see* p.187) or ibuprofen (*see* p.184) to relieve pain. Ibuprofen has an anti-inflammatory effect, which will help reduce swelling and stiffness. Ibuprofen gel, cream, or spray has similar painkilling and anti-inflammatory effects and is applied directly to the affected area.

Counter-irritants (*see* p.180) are creams and gels that produce a tingling sensation in the skin, which soothes pain temporarily.

 ### PRACTICAL TECHNIQUE

Elbow stretches Doing these exercises will warm you up and help to prevent elbow strains.

1 *Hold your forearms and hands straight out in front of you, with your palms downwards. Lightly clench your fists and flex your wrists up and down 10 times.*

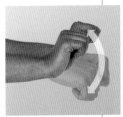

2 *Hold your arms and hands straight out in front of you. Keeping your elbows straight, rotate your hands from palms upwards to palms downwards 10 times.*

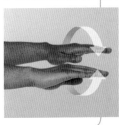

Hip pain

The most common cause of pain and stiffness in the hip is wear and tear due to arthritis. This condition usually affects older people; if you have it, you may feel pain in your thigh, buttock, or groin as well as in your hip. Another cause is bursitis, in which the fluid-filled sac that cushions the hip joint becomes inflamed because of overuse or injury. Bursitis causes pain on the outside of the thigh, close to the hip, that gets worse when you climb stairs or lie on the affected side.

WARNING

Seek immediate medical help if:
- You develop hip pain after an accident or fall
- Walking is difficult, or you cannot put weight on the affected leg
- You have a fever with hip pain

See your doctor first

Make an appointment to see your doctor if you have hip pain to establish the cause.

What you can do yourself

If you have an episode of hip pain, try the following measures to help relieve the discomfort.

- Take a painkiller or apply an ibuprofen preparation. Massaging the hip with a counter-irritant can also be soothing (see DRUG REMEDIES, right).

- Try to keep moving gently, resting your hip and leg whenever you can. Avoid activity that brings on pain or makes it worse.

- If you have bursitis, try applying an ice pack (such as a bag of frozen peas or crushed ice wrapped in a wet towel). Hold in place for about 10 minutes. Reapply 2–3 times a day for the first 48 hours.

- If you have arthritis, hold a covered hot-water bottle or a heated fleece pad on your hip.

- Sleep on a firm mattress. Try not to lie on the hip.

- For arthritis, try a supplement of glucosamine and/or chondroitin (see NATURAL REMEDIES, right).

Seek further medical advice

Arrange to see your doctor if:
- Your hip is not improving after a week, or is getting worse
- You develop pain in other joints

DRUG REMEDIES

Painkillers include paracetamol (see p.187) and ibuprofen (see p.184), which also has an anti-inflammatory effect. Ibuprofen gel, cream, or spray can be applied to the affected area.

Counter-irritants (see p.180) are creams and gels that produce a tingling sensation, which soothes pain temporarily.

NATURAL REMEDIES

Glucosamine and chondroitin (see p.182) occur naturally in joint cartilage. Taking a supplement of either, or both combined, may reduce pain and stiffness and slow the progress of arthritis.

PREVENTION

Avoiding hip pain Once the pain has subsided, take these steps to help prevent recurrences.

- Lose any excess weight, as it puts extra pressure on your hip.
- Cycle or swim regularly to build up the muscles that support your hip joint.

Safe swimming Avoid breaststroke as it can put strain on your hip.

Knee pain

As main weight-bearing joints, knees are easily strained or injured; one or both knees may be painful and may be swollen, warm to the touch, and difficult to move. A sudden twisting movement is a common cause of injury, while inflammation in the joint or in the fluid-filled sacs surrounding it (bursitis) and arthritis are longer-term causes of pain and stiffness.

 See also Sprains and strains, p.160.

> ### WARNING
> Seek immediate medical help if:
> - You have severe knee pain and/or your knee is swollen, red, and hot, and you have a fever
> - You cannot walk after an injury and/or you cannot move your knee

 ## See your doctor first

Make an appointment to see your doctor if:

- You are concerned about a knee injury
- You have pain in other joints and/or you have had knee pain for some time

What you can do yourself

There are several home treatments that will help relieve pain and increase your mobility.

- If you have injured your knee, use the R.I.C.E. procedure (*see* PRACTICAL TECHNIQUE, p.160).

 - Take a painkiller or apply an ibuprofen preparation (*see* DRUG REMEDIES, right).

 - Massaging your knee with a counter-irritant cream or gel may also help soothe the pain (*see* DRUG REMEDIES, right).

- To prevent stiffness, move your knee frequently as far as the pain allows. Gradually increase the range of movement as the pain subsides.

 - If your knee pain is due to arthritis, taking a supplement of glucosamine and/or chondroitin may help in the long term (*see* NATURAL REMEDIES, right).

- Lose weight if you need to do so, because being overweight puts extra stress on the knee joint.

- Wear comfortable shoes with a well-cushioned sole and a low heel.

- Regular exercise, such as walking up stairs or cycling, will strengthen the leg muscles that help to protect and support your joints.

 ### DRUG REMEDIES

Painkillers include paracetamol (*see* p.187) and ibuprofen (*see* p.184), which also has an anti-inflammatory effect. Ibuprofen gel, cream, or spray can be applied to the affected area.

Counter-irritants (*see* p.180) are creams and gels that produce a tingling sensation, which soothes pain temporarily.

 ### NATURAL REMEDIES

Glucosamine and chondroitin (*see* p.182) are naturally occurring substances found in joint cartilage. Taking supplements of either, or a combination of both, may relieve pain and stiffness and slow the progress of arthritis.

Arthritis relief
It may take at least a month for glucosamine and/or chondroitin supplements to have an effect.

Seek further medical advice

Arrange to see your doctor if:

- Pain and swelling from an injury are not subsiding after about 2 days
- The pain is becoming worse
- You develop new symptoms

Leg cramps

A cramp is a painful spasm, usually in one or more calf or foot muscles. The muscle becomes hard and knotted, and hurts if you try to move it. The pain usually lasts for only a few minutes. You may get cramp on waking up or after sitting or lying awkwardly. If you get it during exercise or strenuous work, it is usually due to overusing muscles, heat, dehydration, or salt and mineral loss. Swimmers can get cramp if they become cold and exhausted.

> **WARNING**
>
> Seek urgent medical help if:
> ● You have continuous pain deep in your calf or in a leg vein
> ● Your leg is hot, red, or swollen; turns blue or white; or feels cold

What you can do yourself

Although a cramp will subside on its own, the steps below will help to minimize discomfort.

● If you get cramp during exercise, stop. Gently massage the muscle. If the spasm is in your calf, stretch it. Pull your toes towards your knee, letting your ankle bend. Hold until the muscle relaxes.

● If the cramp occurs while you are in bed, get up and wiggle your foot or walk around. If it persists, try stretching the muscle as above.

● Try heat, particularly for cramp due to swimming. Take a warm bath or shower, then wrap a warm towel around the muscle. Put on warm clothing or cover your leg with a blanket afterwards. For cramp caused by overuse, try an ice pack. Wrap a bag of frozen peas or crushed ice in a wet towel, and hold it on the muscle for 10 minutes.

PREVENTION

Avoiding cramp If you are prone to cramp, the following measures may help to prevent attacks.

● Drink 8 glasses of water a day. Have 1–2 glasses 2 hours before any exercise; ½–1 glass every 15–20 minutes during exercise; and plenty of fluid afterwards.
● Warm up thoroughly before you exercise, and ease off gradually afterwards. Stop when you need to rest.
 ● Do calf-stretching exercises to relieve and prevent cramp (see PRACTICAL TECHNIQUE, right).
● Eat foods rich in potassium, magnesium, and calcium, such as avocados, bananas, oranges, milk, dark-leaved vegetables, wholegrain foods, and nuts.
● Stop smoking; it contributes to the risk of cramp.

PRACTICAL TECHNIQUE

Calf-stretching exercise Try this exercise to relieve an attack of cramp and as a daily routine to prevent further episodes. Do it before and after using your leg muscles for long periods and before going to bed if you are prone to leg cramps at night.

1 Stand about an arm's length from a wall with one leg in front of the other and your hands flat against the wall at shoulder height.

2 Keeping your feet flat on the floor, lean forwards, bending the front knee and pressing the rear heel into the ground. You will feel the calf muscle of the rear leg stretch. Repeat the exercise with the other leg.

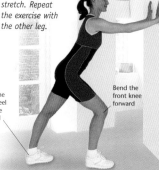

Press the back heel into the ground

Bend the front knee forward

Seek medical advice

Arrange to see your doctor if:

● Cramps are not relieved by these measures, or they become more severe or frequent

Varicose veins

Varicose veins are bluish, distorted veins that bulge beneath the skin, usually on the inside leg, at the back of the calf, or at the ankle. An affected leg may feel heavy, your ankle may swell, and the skin over the veins may be dry and itchy. The problem is more common in women and often runs in families. Pregnancy, constipation, being overweight, or having to stand for long periods increases the risk.

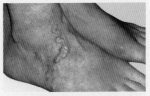

Varicose vein on the ankle and foot

See also Swollen ankles, p.96; Constipation, p.115.

What you can do yourself

Although self-help treatments will not get rid of your varicose veins, they will help to ease the discomfort and stop the veins from getting worse by improving circulation and muscle tone.

- Try to avoid standing for long periods. When this is unavoidable, flex your calf muscles every few minutes and wiggle your toes. If you sit for long periods, get up every 30 minutes and walk around.

- Don't cross your legs when you sit down, as it restricts blood flow in the lower legs.

- When you relax in an armchair, keep your legs raised on a stool or pile of books, but take care not to place anything directly under your knees.

- Wear low-heeled or flat shoes; they make your calf muscles work harder when you walk.

- Don't wear girdles or control-top underwear or tights that constrict your waist or groin and restrict blood flow at the top of your legs. Avoid socks or hold-ups with tight elastic.

- Support stockings may help, especially if you will be standing all day. Put them on first thing in the morning, before your ankles start to swell.

- Use a moisturizing cream if your skin is dry and itchy over the veins (*see* DRUG REMEDIES, right).

- Take care not to knock the fragile skin over a varicose vein, because this may burst the vein and cause severe bleeding.

- Stop smoking; it can contribute to the risk of varicose veins developing.

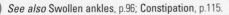

DRUG REMEDIES

Moisturizers (*see* p.186), such as aqueous cream, can be lightly rubbed into the skin over varicose veins to relieve dryness and itching.

PREVENTION

A few lifestyle changes can help to reduce the risk of varicose veins or may help to prevent them getting any worse.

- Lose weight if you are overweight. This will help to relieve the pressure on existing veins and may prevent new varicose veins developing.
- Take regular exercise, such as walking, cycling, and swimming, to boost your circulation.
- To prevent constipation, drink 6–8 glasses of water a day. Include plenty of high-fibre food in your diet such as wholemeal bread; wholegrain cereals; brown rice; vegetables, such as jacket potatoes and baked beans; and fresh fruit.
- Wear support stockings or tights regularly if you are pregnant or if your work involves standing for long periods of time.

 Seek medical advice

Arrange to see your doctor if:

- **Your varicose veins are getting worse or new ones develop**
- **A vein becomes red and feels warm**
- **The skin over a varicose vein becomes discoloured, sore, or weepy**

Swollen ankles

You may develop swollen ankles after a period of inactivity, such as a long car journey or flight, or if you have to spend long periods of time standing up, especially in a hot environment. The swelling is usually caused by a build-up of fluid, as a result of sluggish blood circulation. Your ankles are unlikely to be painful, but you may have an uncomfortable, tight feeling in the skin. The problem can occur with varicose veins, and some women are prone to swollen ankles during pregnancy. Some drugs can contribute to swelling of the ankles, and the problem is sometimes an indication of a heart, kidney, or liver condition.

 See also Varicose veins, p.95.

 ## See your doctor first

Make an appointment to see your doctor if:

- You have pain or tenderness in your calf
- One leg is swollen, with no obvious cause
- You are taking a prescribed medicine that may be causing the problem

What you can do yourself

Try the following measures to reduce swollen ankles or prevent a build-up of fluid.

- To relieve swollen ankles, lie down and prop your legs up 15–30 cm (6–12 in) above the level of your heart. Don't place anything under your knees.

- If you have to stand for long periods, flex your calves every few minutes and wiggle your toes.

- If you are prone to swollen ankles, wear support stockings or tights. Put them on first thing in the morning, before your legs start to swell.

- During long car journeys, stop frequently so that you can stretch your legs.

 - On a long flight, exercise your legs (*see* PRACTICAL TECHNIQUE, right). Try wearing flight socks that use light compression to aid blood flow in the legs.

- Drink 6–8 glasses of water a day to prevent dehydration. Your body will excrete any excess.

- Wear low-heeled or flat shoes; they make the calf muscles work harder than high heels, which improves circulation in the legs.

- Don't wear girdles or control-top underwear or tights. Avoid socks or hold-ups with tight elastic.

 PRACTICAL TECHNIQUE

In-flight exercises During a long flight, do these exercises every 30 minutes to boost blood flow. They will also help prevent the serious disorder deep vein thrombosis ("economy class syndrome"), in which a blood clot develops in the leg.

1 *Starting with your feet flat, keep your heels on the floor and lift your toes as high as you can.*

2 *Now lift your heels high, pressing the balls of your feet into the floor. Do these foot pumps for 30 seconds.*

3 *Stretch one leg out in front of you and circle your foot 8 times in each direction. Change legs and circle the other foot.*

 ## Seek further medical advice

Arrange to see your doctor if:

- Ankle swelling does not subside using the measures described here

Foot pain

Your feet undergo a great deal of wear and pressure. After prolonged standing or walking, they may be aching and swollen, and overactivity can cause pain in the sole or heel, or muscle or tendon strains. Shoes that chafe or squeeze, or sports shoes that do not support the feet, add to the problem. Morton's neuroma (swelling of a nerve between the toe bones) can cause pain in the ball of the foot. Some conditions affecting the whole body, such as gout, diabetes, and arthritis, can also cause foot pain.

 See also **Corns and calluses,** p.42; **Warts and verrucas,** p.43; **Ingrowing toenail,** p.55; **Bunions,** p.98; **Painful heel,** p.99; **Blisters,** p.155.

 ## See your doctor first

Make an appointment to see your doctor if:

- You have diabetes or poor circulation
- Foot pain is due to an injury

What you can do yourself

There are several simple measures that you can take to minimize or relieve foot pain.

- Wear well-fitting shoes in which you can wiggle your toes easily. Avoid shoes with pointed toes or with heels higher than 5 cm (2 in). Alternate pairs of shoes from day to day to give your feet a break.

- Buy new shoes at the end of the day when your feet are likely to be at their largest. Don't buy shoes that are too tight and expect them to stretch.

 - For sports and similar activities, choose shoes that fit comfortably and are suitable for your chosen activity (*see* PRACTICAL TIPS, right).

- Wear trainers to and from work if you have to wear formal shoes at the office.

- For extra support and cushioning, an insole may help. Specialized insoles for sports footwear are available from sports shops.

 - If your feet are hurting, take a painkiller (*see* DRUG REMEDIES, right).

 - Soak aching feet in the bath, but not for too long otherwise the skin will become dry. Afterwards, apply a moisturizer (*see* DRUG REMEDIES, right).

- If the pain is related to a sporting activity, reduce it or stop until the pain has gone.

 ### PRACTICAL TIPS

Choosing sports shoes Your sports shoes should fit comfortably from the start. If you practise a sport regularly, choose shoes designed for that activity; for example, if you run on hard surfaces, you need shoes that support your instep and cushion your heel. When buying new shoes, take the following steps to ensure that they fit correctly.

- Try on the shoes with appropriate sports socks.
- Check that the shoes grip your heels and leave you room to wiggle your toes. Re-lace them yourself so that they apply even pressure to the top of your feet.
- Walk or run a few steps to decide whether or not the shoes are comfortable.

 ### DRUG REMEDIES

Painkillers, such as ibuprofen (*see* p.184) or paracetamol (*see* p.187), will help relieve muscle or joint aches. If the pain does not ease after a few days, stop taking them and arrange to see your doctor.

Moisturizers (*see* p.186) will keep your feet soft and help prevent dry areas from developing. Apply moisturizing cream or lotion just after a bath or shower, while your skin is still moist.

 ## Seek further medical advice

Arrange to see your doctor if:

- You still have foot pain after 2–3 weeks of using the measures suggested here

Bunions

A bunion is a bump at the base of the big toe, caused by a deformity of the joint. If you have bunions, your big toes are pushed inwards, and the protruding toe joints may become red, tender, and swollen. You may also get corns and calluses over the joints if your shoes rub. Bunions tend to run in families. Pressure from narrow shoes contributes to the problem, making bunions more common in women.

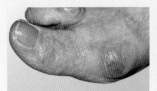

Bunion on right foot

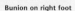 *See also* Corns and calluses, p.42.

 ## See your doctor first

Make an appointment to see your doctor if you have diabetes or suffer from poor circulation.

What you can do yourself

You cannot get rid of a bunion with self-help treatments, but they will help to relieve the discomfort and prevent it from getting worse.

● Put a felt bunion pad over the sore area to reduce pressure and friction. An arch support may also relieve pressure, and shaped rubber pads between your toes may help to keep your big toe in its proper position. Make sure any padding you use does not put pressure on your toes.

 ● If you have to stand or walk for long periods, take a painkiller (*see* DRUG REMEDIES, right).

● Wear properly fitting shoes with a wide toe area, avoiding pointed styles and heels higher than 5 cm (2 in). Buy new shoes at the end of the day.

● Try foot exercises to help prevent a bunion getting worse (*see* PRACTICAL TECHNIQUE, right).

● If a bunion is inflamed, apply an ice pack (such as a bag of frozen peas or crushed ice wrapped in a wet towel) several times a day to reduce the swelling.

 ## Seek further medical advice

Arrange to see your doctor if:

● A bunion becomes inflamed or weepy, or causes continual pain

---

DRUG REMEDIES

Painkillers can be used when your bunion causes severe discomfort. Take ibuprofen (*see* p.184) or paracetamol (*see* p.187) to relieve the pain.

PRACTICAL TECHNIQUE

Foot exercises If you have the beginnings of a bunion, try these exercises to strengthen your foot muscles. They may prevent the bunion getting worse.

1 *Practise picking up a pencil or marble from the floor with your toes. You can do this exercise standing up or sitting down.*

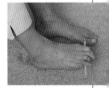

2 *Either standing or sitting, put a small, round, strong glass bottle on the floor and roll each foot in turn over it from toe to heel. Do this 10 times.*

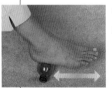

3 *Sitting down, keep your heel on the floor and stretch your toes upwards, fanning them out as far as you can. Then lift and circle each foot 6 times.*

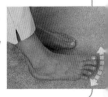

Painful heel

A common cause of heel pain is inflammation of the sole of the foot (plantar fasciitis), which causes severe pain when you first put pressure on your heel in the morning or after sitting. The problem can be due to activities such as jogging, and is worst when you go barefoot or wear thin-soled shoes. Another cause of heel pain is inflammation of the Achilles tendon (Achilles tendinitis), due to overuse or misuse during exercise. Symptoms include a dull ache in the back of the heel and stiffness in the tendon.

> ### WARNING
> Seek immediate medical help if:
> - You feel a "snap" at the back of your ankle during exercise, have severe pain behind your ankle, and/or cannot walk properly
> - Heel pain follows a foot injury

See your doctor first

Make an appointment to see your doctor if you are unsure about the cause of heel pain.

What you can do yourself

Both plantar fasciitis and Achilles tendinitis may be slow to get better. Use the measures below for a few weeks until you see an improvement.

- Try applying an ice pack (such as a bag of frozen peas or crushed ice wrapped in a wet towel) to your heel. Hold it in place for about 10 minutes. Reapply it 2–3 times a day for the first 48 hours.

- If your painful heel is due to plantar fasciitis, massage it for a few minutes in the mornings after a warm bath or shower.

- Take a painkiller such as ibuprofen (*see* DRUG REMEDIES, right).

- Wear shoes with good arch supports and flexible soles. Well-padded sports shoes, laced firmly, will be the most comfortable. If you've strained your Achilles tendon, put a heel pad or piece of foam in your shoe to take the stress off the tendon and make walking less painful.

- Cut back on activities that put pressure on your heel, such as jogging or playing tennis. Try cycling or swimming instead. If you've strained your Achilles tendon, rest completely until the pain has subsided and then begin gentle calf-stretching exercises (*see* PRACTICAL TECHNIQUE, p.94).

DRUG REMEDIES

Painkillers, such as ibuprofen (*see* p.184) or paracetamol (*see* p.187), will reduce the discomfort of a painful heel. If it does not improve after 4–5 days, stop taking the painkiller and see your doctor.

PREVENTION

Protecting your heels You can protect your heels from damage during exercise, and reduce pressure on them, using the following measures.

- Warm up before doing exercise. If your heel starts to hurt, stop; don't try to exercise through the pain.
- If possible, play sports or run on grass or indoor surfaces rather than hard surfaces such as pavements or tarmac.
- Buy sports shoes designed for your chosen activity and lace them firmly (*see* PRACTICAL TIPS: CHOOSING SPORTS SHOES, p.97). At other times, wear well-fitting shoes with good arch supports, cushioned soles, and heels no higher than 5 cm (2 in).
- Practise calf-stretching exercises (*see* PRACTICAL TECHNIQUE, p.94) to increase flexibility and reduce the risk of injury to your tendons.
- If you are overweight, losing weight will help to take some of the strain off your feet.

Seek further medical advice

Arrange to see your doctor if:

- Your heel pain does not subside within a few weeks or becomes more severe

Cold fingers and toes

It is normal for your fingers and toes to react to cold. Some people, though, feel the cold excessively, even if they just put their hands into a refrigerator or hold a cold drink. Poor circulation and underactivity of the thyroid gland can contribute to cold fingers and toes but a more common cause is Raynaud's, in which tiny blood vessels in the fingers (and sometimes the toes) go into spasm, usually in response to cold. The fingers or toes go white and cold, then blue. As the blood returns, they go red and may tingle, throb, or feel numb or painful. Raynaud's can also be caused by working with vibrating tools such as chainsaws, some prescribed drugs, and stress, or it may occur as a symptom of diseases affecting blood vessels or joints.

 ## See your doctor first

Make an appointment to see your doctor if your fingers or toes are exceptionally sensitive to cold, to establish the cause.

What you can do yourself

If your fingers and toes are very sensitive to cold, try these steps to reduce the severity of symptoms.

- Try to avoid handling cold objects. Use mittens or a towel to remove food from a freezer or fridge. Use a cup holder when drinking a cold drink.

- Stop smoking: nicotine causes narrowing of the blood vessels and contributes to Raynaud's.

- Cut down on caffeinated drinks such as coffee.

- Keeping your body warm helps the circulation to your hands and feet. Dress warmly when you go out in cold weather (*see* PRACTICAL TIPS, right).

- If your fingers turn white and numb, swing your arms in large circles, clenching and unclenching your hands. Wiggle your toes to increase blood flow. Use hot-air dryers in toilets to warm your hands, or soak fingers and toes in warm water.

- Make sure your bed clothes are warm. An electric blanket may help, as will wearing socks in bed.

 ## Seek further medical advice

Arrange to see your doctor if:

- Your symptoms are persistent or getting worse
- You develop any new, unexplained symptoms, such as joint pains

PRACTICAL TIPS

Dressing to stay warm Put on several thin layers of clothing to trap heat next to your skin; thermal underwear may help.

- Wear a hat and warm your hands before putting on gloves (or mittens, which are even warmer). Try battery-heated gloves or hand heating aids.
- Wear warm socks and put padding in your shoes or boots. Avoid tight-fitting footwear and clothes because they restrict blood circulation.

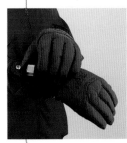

Heated gloves
These gloves are useful if you have to be out of doors for long spells in cold weather. They are powered by a battery in a pouch in the wrist and stay warm for 5–6 hours.

PREVENTION

Preventing attacks If you regularly have cold fingers and toes, a few lifestyle changes can help to prevent or reduce the frequency of attacks.

- Take regular exercise to stimulate the circulation.
- If your problem is triggered by stress, practising some deep breathing exercises and muscle relaxation techniques (*see* PRACTICAL TECHNIQUES, pp.20–21) may help you reduce it.
- Avoid using vibrating tools if this is a trigger.

CHEST AND ABDOMINAL PROBLEMS

Hiccups

Everyone has an occasional bout of hiccups – short, sharp intakes of air caused by repeated, involuntary spasms of your diaphragm. Although they often occur for no apparent reason, common causes include overeating or eating too fast; eating spicy, very hot, or very cold food; drinking fizzy drinks; or drinking alcohol. Smoking heavily, or emotional factors such as nervousness or shock, can bring on an attack of hiccups, as can a sudden change in temperature. Hiccups usually last for no more than a few minutes. Bouts that last more than a few days can be a sign of illness, and may also lead to difficulty in sleeping and weight loss.

What you can do yourself

Attacks of hiccups disappear of their own accord but if you need to get rid of them quickly, try some of these home remedies.

● Hold your breath for as long as you can, or breathe in and out quickly. Alternatively, breathe into a paper bag (*see* PRACTICAL TECHNIQUE, right).

● Sip iced water, or chew and swallow pieces of crushed ice, for 10–15 minutes.

● Eat a dry piece of bread or a cracker.

● Place a teaspoonful of granulated sugar on the back of your tongue and swallow it.

● Suck on a slice of lemon soaked in Angostura bitters, or sip a small amount of vinegar.

● Pull hard on your tongue, or touch the back of your tongue with your finger or a cotton bud.

● Sit on a chair or on the floor and pull your knees up towards your chest while leaning forwards.

● Have someone else startle you unexpectedly. This is sometimes enough to stop a hiccup attack.

Seek medical advice

Arrange to see your doctor if:

● A bout of hiccups has lasted for longer than 24 hours
● You get frequent bouts of hiccups

PRACTICAL TECHNIQUE

Rebreathing Hold a brown paper bag (not a plastic bag) over your nose and mouth, and breathe in and out of it forcefully 10 times. Exhaled air contains higher levels of carbon dioxide than normal, and rebreathing it from a bag may help to relax your diaphragm and stop the hiccups.

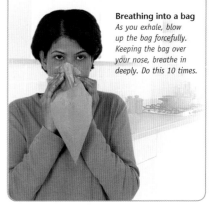

Breathing into a bag
As you exhale, blow up the bag forcefully. Keeping the bag over your nose, breathe in deeply. Do this 10 times.

Coughing

The most common cause of a cough is irritation or inflammation in your lungs or throat due to a cold or flu, a chest infection, or asthma. Irritants such as tobacco smoke, dust, and pollen can make you cough, as can post-nasal drip (mucus from the nose dripping down the back of the throat), or regurgitation of stomach acid in heartburn. Some people have a nervous cough that becomes a habit. A cough may be simply dry, tickly, and irritating, or it may bring up mucus (a "productive" cough). Some prescribed drugs cause coughing. Occasionally, however, a cough is a symptom of a serious illness such as cancer.

 See also Blocked or runny nose, p.77; Acute bronchitis, p.104; Heartburn, p.107.

 See your doctor first

Arrange to see your doctor promptly if:

- You have breathing problems or chest pain
- You cough up blood or discoloured mucus
- You are feverish and sweating
- You are losing weight
- You are taking prescribed medicine that may be causing the cough, such as certain drugs to control blood pressure

What you can do yourself

There are several things that you can do to help control a cough and to support any treatment recommended by your doctor.

- Drink at least 8 glasses of fluids a day. Include warm drinks such as soup and herbal tea, which help to thin mucus and make it easier to cough up.

- To soothe your throat, try a warm honey and lemon drink (*see* NATURAL REMEDIES, p.30).

 - Normally, you shouldn't suppress a cough, as it clears the airway. However, if you have a dry, tickly cough that makes it difficult for you to sleep, try a cough suppressant (*see* DRUG REMEDIES, right).

- Warm, moist air can loosen mucus and soothe a cough. Use a humidifier, or place a bowl of water by a radiator, or hang a wet towel close to it. Steam inhalation may help (*see* PRACTICAL TECHNIQUE, p.79).

- Raising the head of the bed or sleeping on extra pillows may help to ease a cough at night.

- Avoid smoky or dusty environments and being near people who are smoking. If you smoke, stop.

DRUG REMEDIES

Cough suppressants (*see* p.180) containing pholcodine or dextromethorphan will help to control a dry cough that keeps you awake at night or makes it difficult for you to work. Don't take cough suppressants with alcohol.

If you have a productive cough (one that brings up mucus), it is best not to take any cough mixture because coughing helps to clear the mucus and irritants from the airways. (Expectorant medicines for loosening mucus are usually of little value.)

Using suppressants
Limit your use of cough suppressants during the day, because they may cause drowsiness.

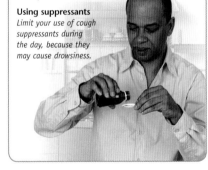

 Seek further medical advice

Arrange to see your doctor if:

- The cough is getting worse, or it has not begun to get better after a week
- You are becoming exhausted by coughing
- The mucus becomes green, yellow, or bloodstained

Wheezing

Wheezing is a high-pitched whistling as you breathe out. Your chest may feel tight and you may find it hard to breathe. The most common cause is asthma; attacks are often an allergic reaction to inhaled substances such as dust, or are due to stress, cold air, or exercise. Other causes of wheezing include chest infection; tobacco smoke; a severe allergic reaction; or a heart or lung problem.

 See also Hay fever, p.80; Anaphylactic shock, p.159.

> **WARNING**
>
> Seek immediate medical help if:
> - You begin to wheeze suddenly or your lips or tongue turn blue
> - You feel frightened by your shortness of breath

See your doctor first

Arrange to see your doctor promptly if you have a wheezy chest. Check if you are taking drugs that may cause wheezing, such as anti-inflammatory painkillers or beta-blockers.

What you can do yourself

These measures will help to relieve or prevent asthma attacks, or wheezing due to other causes, and support any treatment from your doctor.

- When an asthma attack begins, try to keep calm and breathe slowly. Sit in a comfortable position; you may find it helpful to lean forward and rest your arms on a table or the back of a chair.

- If you use an asthma inhaler, keep it with you at all times and use it as directed. Keep extra inhalers at home and at work or school.

- If stress makes wheezing worse, try practising deep breathing and muscle relaxation exercises (*see* PRACTICAL TECHNIQUES, pp.20–21). You can also use them to calm yourself during an attack.

- Regular exercise, such as walking and swimming in a heated pool, can improve symptoms and keep you fit, as long as they don't make wheezing worse.

- Keep out of cold air; if you have to go out, wrap a scarf loosely around your face to warm the air as you breathe. When the air pollution level is high, stay indoors and keep doors and windows closed.

- Avoid smoky or dusty environments and allergens that might provoke an asthma attack (*see* PREVENTION, right). If you smoke, stop.

PREVENTION

Reducing allergens in the home
Many people with asthma are allergic to the droppings of house dust mites. Other triggers include mould, fur and dander (flakes of skin) from pets, and household chemicals. Take these steps to reduce triggers.

- Dust surfaces with a damp cloth and try to reduce clutter in your home. Don't have too many soft toys for a child with asthma. Every 2 weeks, put them in a bag in the freezer for 6 hours, or through a hot wash.
- Use pillows and duvets with synthetic fillings, and covers that protect users from house dust mites. Buy a mattress cover that fits over the whole mattress, not just the top. Wash bed linen weekly at 60°C (140°F). Clean curtains regularly or replace them with blinds.
- Replace carpets with wooden or vinyl flooring, if possible, or choose short-pile synthetic carpets.
- Vacuum regularly; use a high-powered cleaner with a filter. Ask someone else to empty the machine.
- Make sure that your home is well ventilated. Keep kitchen and bathroom doors closed to prevent damp from spreading. Treat any mould on tiles, shower curtains, and bathroom windows with a weak bleach solution. Avoid using chemicals with strong fumes.
- If you're allergic to a pet, you may have to give it up. If you can't, keep the pet out of your bedroom completely and out of main living areas as much as possible. Have your pet groomed or bathed regularly.

Seek further medical advice

Arrange to see your doctor if:

- You cannot control asthma or other wheezing attacks using these measures

Acute bronchitis

Acute bronchitis is an infection of the airways in the lungs. It causes an irritating, persistent cough that sometimes produces thick or coloured mucus (phlegm). You may also have wheezing, a fever, headache, and aches and pains. The illness is usually caused by a virus and often follows on from a cold. If you are otherwise healthy, it is not normally serious; you should be feeling a lot better within a few days, although the cough may linger for 3–4 weeks. You may be prone to bronchitis if you smoke or if you are exposed to pollution. People who have lung disease may have several attacks each winter.

➡ *See also* Coughing, p.102; Wheezing, p.103.

 ## See your doctor first

Make an appointment to see your doctor if:

- You have a persistent cough and are elderly
- You have a lung condition such as asthma, or a heart problem such as heart failure
- You have difficulty breathing and chest tightness, or you are coughing up thick green, yellow, or bloodstained mucus

What you can do yourself

The following steps will help to relieve symptoms while the infection is clearing up.

- Get plenty of rest for the first few days of an attack, although you don't need to stay in bed.

- Drink at least 8 glasses of fluids a day. Warm fluids, such as soup, may be comforting.

- To soothe an irritated throat, try a warm honey and lemon drink (*see* NATURAL REMEDIES, p.30).

 - Take a painkiller to reduce a temperature (*see* DRUG REMEDIES, right).

- Don't try to suppress a cough that produces mucus, as this is the body's way of clearing the airways. If you have a dry cough, however, try a cough suppressant (*see* DRUG REMEDIES, right).

- Warm, moist air loosens mucus. Use a humidifier, place a bowl of water beside a radiator to moisten the air, or sit in the bathroom while you run a bath and inhale the steam. A steam inhalation may also be helpful (*see* PRACTICAL TECHNIQUE, p.79).

- If you smoke, stop. Avoid smoky atmospheres.

 ### DRUG REMEDIES

Painkillers such as paracetamol (*see* p.187) or ibuprofen (*see* p.184) will reduce your temperature and help you feel more comfortable.

Cough suppressants (*see* p.180) containing pholcodine or dextromethorphan can help relieve a dry cough that is keeping you awake at night. Some also contain sedating antihistamines (*see* p.178) to help you sleep. Don't take suppressants with alcohol.

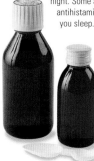

Sedative medicine
Cough suppressants are usually available as liquids. Some brands are useful at bedtime, because they help you sleep.

 ## Seek further medical advice

Arrange to see your doctor if:

- You are not feeling better after 3–4 days, or the cough has not subsided within 3–4 weeks
- Breathing becomes more difficult, or you develop chest pains
- You have recurrent episodes of bronchitis

Palpitations

If you have palpitations you are suddenly aware of your heartbeat, which may feel normal, fast, or irregular. This is a common problem. Causes include exercise, excitement, stress, anxiety, and stimulants such as caffeine and nicotine. Palpitations usually occur with no other symptoms and last for a few seconds or minutes. They are normally harmless, but may be a cause for concern if they occur without obvious cause or with other symptoms, or are prolonged.

> **WARNING**
>
> Seek immediate medical help if:
> - You have palpitations and are sweaty, short of breath, have chest pain, or feel dizzy or faint
> - You suffer from an existing heart condition

 See also Panic attacks, p.24.

See your doctor first

Arrange to see your doctor urgently if you have a prolonged episode of palpitations and/or frequent missed heartbeats.

What you can do yourself

If you experience occasional palpitations, try the following to help identify and deal with the cause.

- Keep a diary, noting when you have palpitations and any food or drink, exercise, stress, or other possible triggers that you have at the same time.

- If you are feeling stressed, try practising some deep breathing and muscle relaxation exercises (*see* PRACTICAL TECHNIQUES, pp.20–21).

- Try to get plenty of sleep. Exhaustion from lack of sleep can cause or aggravate palpitations.

 - Reduce your intake of drinks containing caffeine (*see* PRACTICAL TIPS, right). Avoid using over-the-counter stimulant tablets containing caffeine.

- Before using cough or cold remedies, check the labels carefully. Some contain decongestant drugs that can cause palpitations.

- Reduce your intake of alcohol; excessive drinking is a common cause of palpitations.

- Try to give up smoking, as nicotine can speed up your heartbeat and lead to palpitations.

- Don't take illegal stimulants such as solvents, amphetamines, or cocaine, because all of these substances can cause palpitations.

PRACTICAL TIPS

Drinking less caffeine Drinks containing caffeine include coffee, tea, and cola. Reduce your intake to 2 cups a day or less, but cut down gradually; if you do it too rapidly, you may get headaches.

- Have drinks that are lower in caffeine. For example, have decaffeinated coffee, or instant coffee (which has half as much caffeine as freshly brewed coffee).
- Make instant coffee with half regular and half decaffeinated coffee.
- If you drink tea, brew it for less time than normal.
- Drink caffeine-free drinks such as water, fruit juice, and herbal tea.
- Check soft drink labels. Some colas, citrus-flavoured drinks, and energy drinks have high caffeine levels.

Seek further medical advice

Arrange to see your doctor if:

- You have recurrent episodes of palpitations despite trying to cut out possible triggers
- You develop other symptoms, such as weight loss or tiredness

Indigestion

Indigestion is stomach discomfort that usually occurs after meals, often with nausea, belching, and bloating. It is commonly caused by overindulgence in food or drink, and stress, tiredness, or being overweight can aggravate symptoms. Sometimes indigestion is due to a serious disorder such as a stomach ulcer or gallstones, or is a side effect of medicines such as iron or certain antibiotics.

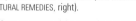 *See also* Heartburn, opposite; Bloating and flatulence, p.108.

> **WARNING**
> Seek immediate medical help if:
> ● You also have chest pain, sweating, and shortness of breath
> ● You are vomiting blood or passing black stools

 ## See your doctor first

Make an appointment to see your doctor if:

● You have severe pain
● Indigestion does not seem related to eating
● You are losing weight without trying
● You are over 45 and have only recently developed indigestion

What you can do yourself

Most bouts of mild indigestion can be dealt with simply by lifestyle adjustments and home remedies.

● Avoid foods or drinks that trigger symptoms.

● Don't exercise for at least an hour after eating.

● If stress contributes to indigestion, try some methods that help to reduce it (*see* pp.20–21).

● Stop smoking, as this may aggravate symptoms.

 ● Take an antacid, an H2-blocker, or a combined H2-blocker and antacid to relieve symptoms (*see* DRUG REMEDIES, right).

● Eat at regular times. You're less likely to get indigestion if you eat smaller meals more often. Eat slowly, chewing your food thoroughly.

● Avoid taking aspirin or ibuprofen for pain, as they can irritate the stomach. Paracetamol (*see* p.187) may be a more suitable alternative.

 ● Try a herbal tea to soothe your stomach (*see* NATURAL REMEDIES, right).

● If you are overweight, try to lose weight gradually.

DRUG REMEDIES

Antacids (*see* p.177) can relieve indigestion by neutralizing acid in the stomach. Some antacids are combined with dimeticone (also known as simeticone) or an H2-blocker (*see* p.182).

H2-blockers (*see* p.182) reduce acid produced by the stomach. Try a short course (not more than 2 weeks) of ranitidine, famotidine, or a combined H2-blocker and antacid if antacids alone are not effective.

Antacids
Liquids are more effective; tablets may be more convenient.

 ### NATURAL REMEDIES

Herbal tea (*see* p.183) made with peppermint, camomile, gentian, or fennel may help to relieve symptoms of indigestion.

Seek further medical advice

Arrange to see your doctor if:

● Your symptoms become worse
● Symptoms are not improving after a week or two
● You have recurrent indigestion

Heartburn

Heartburn is a burning feeling that starts in your lower chest and stomach and may rise to your throat. You may have a bitter taste in your mouth, and feel sick and bloated. Some people have a dry cough, especially at night. Heartburn often occurs after a heavy meal, and is more likely if you lie down or bend over. It is due to acid reflux, in which stomach acid leaks into the gullet.

See also Indigestion, opposite page.

WARNING

Seek immediate medical help if:
- You have prolonged chest pain, sweating, and shortness of breath
- You are vomiting blood or passing black stools
- You have difficulty swallowing

See your doctor first

Make an appointment to see your doctor if:

- You have severe pain
- Heartburn does not seem related to eating
- You are losing weight without trying
- You are over 45 and have only recently developed heartburn

What you can do yourself

Try the following measures to relieve heartburn.

- Avoid foods that trigger heartburn; stop smoking.

- Try taking an antacid, H2-blocker, or proton pump inhibitor (*see* DRUG REMEDIES, right).

- Eat small, regular meals rather than occasional big meals. Don't eat within 2 or 3 hours of bedtime.

- Avoid painkillers or cold remedies that contain aspirin or ibuprofen; they may aggravate heartburn.

- Try a soothing herbal tea to help relieve heartburn (*see* NATURAL REMEDIES, opposite page).

- Sleep with your head raised to help prevent acid reflux (*see* PRACTICAL TIP, right).

- If you are overweight, try to lose weight gradually.

Seek further medical advice

Arrange to see your doctor if:

- Your symptoms become worse, or do not improve after a week or two
- You are getting recurrent bouts of heartburn

DRUG REMEDIES

Antacids (*see* p.177) neutralize acid in the stomach, providing quick relief for occasional, mild episodes of heartburn. Choose an antacid containing an alginate. Antacids are more effective in liquid form than as tablets.

H2-blockers (*see* p.182) and **proton pump inhibitors** (*see* p.187) work by reducing acid production in the stomach. Ask your pharmacist to recommend a suitable medication.

PRACTICAL TIP

Sleep with your head raised
To help prevent stomach acid leaking back into your gullet at night, keep your head higher than your body. Prop up the head of your bed 10–15 cm (4–6 in). If you take naps during the day, sleep upright in a chair.

Raising the bed head
Sturdy, solid objects, such as bricks or pieces of wood, placed under the head of the bed help to keep your head raised.

Bloating and flatulence

A bloated abdomen and flatulence (wind) are common complaints, caused by a build-up of excess gas in your digestive system. You may also experience sharp pains and rumbling noises in your abdomen. Most cases of bloating and flatulence are due to food, particularly foods such as beans and cabbage, which produce gas as they are digested. Eating too fast can also cause excessive wind. Certain people find that milk, food additives, or wheat flour can produce symptoms. Sometimes, bloating and flatulence are due to a bowel disorder such as irritable bowel syndrome.

 See also Irritable bowel syndrome, p.111; Food intolerance, p.113.

See your doctor first

Make an appointment to see your doctor if you also have other bowel symptoms, such as constipation, diarrhoea, blood in your stools, nausea, vomiting, or continual or recurrent abdominal pains.

What you can do yourself

Try these measures to prevent a build-up of wind or to treat bloating and flatulence.

- Try to identify and cut down on any foods that cause problems. The worst offenders include cabbage, cauliflower, Brussels sprouts, onions, garlic, prunes, raisins, beans, and spicy foods.

- You may develop wind or bloating if you add high-fibre foods to your diet too quickly. Reduce your intake, then increase it gradually over 2–3 weeks.

- Eat and drink slowly, and chew food thoroughly. You may find it helps to eat several small meals a day instead of one or two large ones.

- Cut down on beer and fizzy drinks; chewing gum; smoking; and the artificial sweeteners sorbitol and mannitol (found in some sugar-free sweet foods). All of these things may contribute to flatulence.

 - Preparations containing dimeticone can be used to treat flatulence (*see* DRUG REMEDIES, right).

 - Try using charcoal tablets or biscuits to reduce excess wind (*see* DRUG REMEDIES, right).

 - Try drinking a herbal tea to relieve symptoms (*see* NATURAL REMEDIES, right).

DRUG REMEDIES

Dimeticone (*see* FLATULENCE RELIEF, p.182) helps to disperse excess wind. It is usually combined with an antacid as an indigestion remedy.

Charcoal tablets and biscuits (*see* FLATULENCE RELIEF, p.182) help wind in the digestive system to pass easily out of the body.

NATURAL REMEDIES

Herbal teas (*see* p.183) made with camomile, peppermint, fennel, or gentian may help to calm a bloated stomach and relieve excess wind.

Soothing tea
Sip a soothing herbal tea to help relieve digestive problems.

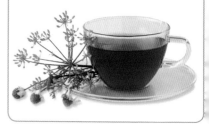

Seek further medical advice

Arrange to see your doctor if bloating and flatulence persist after 2 weeks or new symptoms develop.

Nausea and vomiting

There are many reasons for nausea. The mere sight or smell of something unpleasant, or a food you dislike, may trigger sweating and queasiness. Anxiety and travel sickness are also common causes. Nausea doesn't always lead to vomiting; if it does, it is often due to gastroenteritis (an infection), food poisoning, or excess alcohol. Morning sickness is common in early pregnancy, and migraine sufferers may vomit during attacks. Nausea and vomiting are usually short-lived, but repeated vomiting may dehydrate you.

> **WARNING**
>
> Seek immediate medical help if nausea and vomiting follow a head injury or are accompanied by:
> - Blood in the vomit
> - Severe headache or stiff neck
> - Severe abdominal pain

See your doctor first

Arrange to see your doctor if you can't establish the cause of your nausea or vomiting.

What you can do yourself

Try these measures to help you recover quickly from nausea and/or vomiting and prevent dehydration.

- If you feel nauseous, open a window or step outside for a few minutes to get some fresh air.

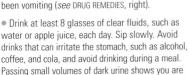

- Take an oral rehydration preparation if you have been vomiting (*see* DRUG REMEDIES, right).

- Drink at least 8 glasses of clear fluids, such as water or apple juice, each day. Sip slowly. Avoid drinks that can irritate the stomach, such as alcohol, coffee, and cola, and avoid drinking during a meal. Passing small volumes of dark urine shows you are becoming dehydrated and need to drink more.

- If you can, eat small, frequent meals. Eat slowly. Start with bland foods such as boiled rice, pasta, chicken soup, or dry toast. Avoid spicy and greasy foods and very hot or very cold foods and drinks.

- Try to rest after meals; sit in a chair or propped up in bed (lying flat may make you feel worse). Don't move around too much, as this can lead to vomiting.

- Avoid strong odours such as perfumes, as they can provoke vomiting.

- Taking ginger (*see* NATURAL REMEDIES, right) may relieve nausea, especially motion sickness.

- If you have morning sickness, keep plain biscuits by your bed and eat one just before you get up.

DRUG REMEDIES

Oral rehydration preparations (*see* p.186) replace salts, sugar, and minerals that have been lost from your body through vomiting. They are available as sachets of powder, which you mix with a recommended amount of drinking water. Have them instead of, or in addition to, regular drinks.

NATURAL REMEDIES

Ginger (*see* p.182) can be soothing during a bout of nausea and can be a useful treatment for motion sickness (*see* p.110). You can take ginger root capsules; alternatively, eat some pieces of crystallized or raw ginger, add powdered ginger to a glass of fruit juice, or make ginger tea.

Seek further medical advice

Arrange to see your doctor if:

- Your nausea or vomiting doesn't start to subside within 24 hours
- You develop any other symptoms
- You are taking regular medication, such as the contraceptive pill, because vomiting may reduce its effectiveness

Motion sickness

If you suffer from motion sickness or travel sickness, you will have feelings of nausea and dizziness, and possibly also a headache, whenever you travel by car, ship, train, or plane. If the motion continues, you begin to feel worse and may break out in a sweat, breathe rapidly and shallowly, turn pale, and vomit. Motion sickness occurs when your brain receives conflicting messages from the balance organs inside the ears and from the eyes. Some people are more susceptible to motion sickness than others, and anxiety can contribute to the problem. Children are generally more prone to the condition than adults.

What you can do yourself

There are several measures that help to prevent or minimize motion sickness. Plan how to put them into effect before you start your journey.

- Before you travel, eat a little bland food. Avoid alcohol and fizzy drinks before and during travel.

- Try taking travel sickness pills before travelling (*see* DRUG REMEDIES, right).

- On board a vehicle, try to choose a position with the least motion. In a plane, sit halfway down, by a window overlooking the wings. In a ship, sit in the middle, or stay on deck if you can. If you are below deck or in an enclosed cabin, try to sleep as much as you can. In a train, sit by a window, facing the direction of travel. In a car, sit in a front seat.

- Make sure that you have access to fresh air. Avoid strong odours and cigarette smoke.

- In a car or train, focus on the horizon or something in the distance in the direction of travel. Avoid reading, writing, or looking down.

- Eating some ginger may help to relieve nausea (*see* NATURAL REMEDIES, right).

- You may find that travelling at night reduces sickness, particularly if you manage to sleep.

- If anxiety plays a part, try exercises to control your breathing (*see* PRACTICAL TECHNIQUE, p.20).

- Try acupressure bands. They are thought to relieve nausea by stimulating a point on the wrist.

- If your child has motion sickness, use a booster seat so that he or she can look out of the window. Distract your child with music, a story tape or CD, or games that involve looking for things ahead.

DRUG REMEDIES

Travel sickness pills (*see* p.189) contain anti-nausea drugs such as hyoscine, or antihistamines, such as meclizine or promethazine, which help to control symptoms. Take them before you start a journey. They may make you drowsy, so don't drive. They may also increase the effects of alcohol, so avoid alcoholic drinks once you have taken them.

NATURAL REMEDIES

Ginger (*see* p.182) has been shown to reduce symptoms of travel sickness. Take ginger root capsules an hour or two before you start a journey. Alternatively, try nibbling a small slice of fresh ginger or crystallized ginger, or taking ½ –1 teaspoon of powdered ginger in fruit juice. A child may prefer a ginger biscuit.

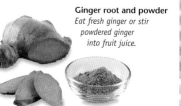

Ginger root and powder
Eat fresh ginger or stir powdered ginger into fruit juice.

⊕ Seek medical advice

Arrange to see your doctor if:

- You still have motion sickness symptoms a day or two after travel
- You have symptoms such as nausea and dizziness when you are not travelling

Irritable bowel syndrome

Symptoms of irritable bowel syndrome (IBS) vary. The most common are bloating, abdominal pain, and cramps, which ease after you pass wind or a bowel motion. You may have loose stools or be constipated, or alternate between the two; notice mucus in your stools; and have the feeling that your bowel has not emptied after a bowel movement. You may feel full more quickly than normal during meals. Other symptoms include nausea, back pain, frequent urination, and headaches. Although symptoms are intermittent, IBS may last for years. The cause is not known, but sensitivity to certain foods, bowel infection, and stress can trigger attacks.

 See also **Stress**, pp.20–21; **Bloating and flatulence**, p.108; **Constipation**, p.115; **Diarrhoea**, p.116.

See your doctor first

Make an appointment to see your doctor if you think you have IBS. Other causes need to be ruled out, because symptoms of IBS are similar to those of more serious bowel conditions.

What you can do yourself

Try the following changes to your diet and lifestyle to see what works best for you.

● Keep a diary for 2 or 3 weeks, noting what you eat and drink and when attacks occur, to identify any triggers. Common triggers for IBS include dairy products, wheat, citrus fruits, alcohol, and coffee.

● Eat and drink slowly, and chew food thoroughly. It may help to eat several small meals a day. Eat at regular times and don't skip meals.

 ● If constipation is a problem, gradually add more fibre to your diet, such as cereals, wholemeal bread, brown rice, beans, fruit, and vegetables. Avoid unprocessed bran as it can make symptoms worse. Try fibre supplements (*see* DRUG REMEDIES, right).

● If you have diarrhoea, cut down on tea, coffee, cola, alcohol, and fatty foods, and stop smoking, to avoid irritating the bowels. Drink 6–8 glasses of water a day and avoid fizzy drinks.

● Walk, cycle, or swim for 20–30 minutes a day to help reduce stress and regulate the bowels.

● If stress triggers IBS, practise exercises to help you relax (*see* PRACTICAL TECHNIQUES, pp.20–21).

● If lifestyle changes don't help, try antispasmodic or antidiarrhoeal drugs (*see* DRUG REMEDIES, right).

DRUG REMEDIES

Fibre supplements (*see* LAXATIVES, p.185) contain fibre derived from plants. They can help if you are prone to constipation and are finding it difficult to include extra fibre in your diet. Consult your doctor before taking fibre supplements.

Antispasmodic drugs (*see* p.178) contain alverine, mebeverine, peppermint oil, or hyoscine. These medicines work by relaxing the bowel muscle, helping to relieve pain and bloating.

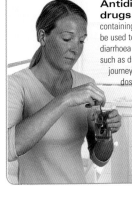

Antidiarrhoeal drugs (*see* p.177) containing loperamide can be used to help control diarrhoea for a limited time, such as during a long car journey. Take the lowest dose that helps.

Taking fibre supplements
Mix the fibre supplement in half a glass of water and drink it immediately.

Seek further medical advice

Arrange to see your doctor if:

● Your symptoms worsen or do not subside after 2 weeks of following the self-help measures given on this page
● You develop new symptoms

Hernia

A hernia is a lump in the groin or, less commonly, at the navel, that tends to disappear when you lie flat. In men, a hernia may appear in the scrotum. You may have no other symptoms, or may feel pain or a dragging sensation. Hernias occur when part of the intestine pushes through a weak spot in your abdominal muscles. They are often due to increased pressure in the abdomen as a result of activities such as heavy lifting, coughing, sneezing, or straining on the toilet. Being overweight makes you more susceptible.

> **WARNING**
>
> Seek urgent medical help if:
> • You have a hernia that you can't gently push back in and/or you have heat and tenderness over the lump; nausea and vomiting; severe abdominal pain; and constipation

See your doctor first

Arrange to see your doctor to confirm that you have a hernia and to discuss treatment.

What you can do yourself

A hernia usually needs surgery, but there are several things you can do that will support treatment from your doctor.

 • If your work involves heavy lifting, try to arrange lighter duties. Once you are better, take care with lifting heavy objects (*see* PREVENTION, right).

• Eat a high-fibre diet with plenty of fruit, vegetables, and wholemeal bread, and drink 6–8 glasses of water a day; this will help keep your bowel movements regular. Avoid straining when you are on the toilet.

• Stop smoking, because a smoker's cough puts pressure on a hernia.

• Lose any excess weight, because the weight puts a strain on your abdominal wall.

• Wearing a groin support is of only limited value unless the device has been fitted properly on the advice of a doctor.

Seek further medical help

Arrange to see your doctor again if:

• The hernia gets larger and more painful while you're waiting for treatment

PREVENTION

Lifting heavy objects The following technique may help prevent another hernia, particularly if your job involves heavy manual work. If an object feels too heavy, don't try to lift or move it without a lifting aid, wheel base, or trolley.

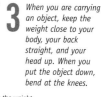

1 *When you lift a heavy object, bend your knees (not your back) and use your leg muscles to provide the lifting power. Squat close to the object and grasp it at the base.*

Keep your back straight and avoid twisting

2 *Straighten your knees and push yourself up with your leg muscles in one smooth movement.*

3 *When you are carrying an object, keep the weight close to your body, your back straight, and your head up. When you put the object down, bend at the knees.*

Keep the weight balanced over your thighs and feet

Food intolerance

If you have symptoms such as bloating, abdominal pain, diarrhoea, or nausea each time you eat a certain food, you may be "intolerant" of it, or unable to digest it properly. The most likely triggers are dairy products and cereals (such as wheat). Food intolerance is distinct from food allergy, which is less common but in some people can cause a life-threatening reaction called anaphylactic shock.

See also Bloating and flatulence, p.108; Diarrhoea, p.116; Anaphylactic shock, p.159.

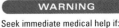

WARNING

Seek immediate medical help if:
- You develop breathing difficulties, swelling of your lips and tongue, and a rash within a few minutes of eating a suspect food

See your doctor first

Make an appointment to see your doctor if:

- You think you may be intolerant of wheat, rye, barley, and possibly oats (gluten intolerance, also called coeliac disease) or of milk and other dairy products (lactose intolerance)
- You have symptoms such as weight loss

What you can do yourself

The following advice will help you identify and treat mild food intolerance; use it alongside any advice from your doctor.

- Try to identify the food causing your symptoms (*see* PRACTICAL TECHNIQUE, right).

- If your doctor has diagnosed lactose intolerance, avoid dairy products. Try soya milk or other milk substitutes, which are now available in many supermarkets. Check for hidden lactose in foods such as biscuits. You may also wish to try a lactase supplement (*see* DRUG REMEDIES, right).

- If you are diagnosed as having gluten intolerance (coeliac disease), cut out cereals, bread, pasta, cakes, and biscuits. Check for hidden gluten in processed foods such as ice cream and tinned soup; sweets; and some medicines. Many supermarkets and health food shops sell gluten-free pastas, breads, and other foods.

- Check labels on food packaging for the food or additive to which you're intolerant. This may not always be obvious: for example, "casein" is milk protein, and "albumin" is egg white.

PRACTICAL TECHNIQUE

Elimination diet If you think you may have a food intolerance, take these steps to find the trigger.

- Keep a diary for 2–3 weeks, noting what you eat and drink and how much, and when symptoms occur. (Symptoms can develop from a few hours to a few days after exposure to a trigger substance.)
- Exclude a suspect substance from your diet for a week or two. If symptoms return when you reintroduce the item, you may be intolerant of it.
- If you find a specific trigger, avoid it. However, if you think you are affected by a whole group of foods, such as dairy or wheat products, see your doctor first.

DRUG REMEDIES

Lactase supplements (*see* p.184) help to break down lactose in dairy foods. They are useful if you are lactose intolerant and find it difficult to limit your milk intake, or if you develop symptoms after having even small amounts of dairy products.

Seek further medical advice

Arrange to see your doctor if:

- Your symptoms don't improve after using the measures described above
- You develop any new symptoms, such as weight loss

Food poisoning

Most attacks of food poisoning are due to poor hygiene, cooking, or food storage, which allows bacteria or viruses in contaminated food to multiply. The most commonly affected foods are seafood, dairy products, and undercooked eggs and poultry. Symptoms of food poisoning include nausea, vomiting, diarrhoea, and cramps in the abdomen, and, sometimes, fever, headache, and dizziness.

WARNING

Seek immediate medical help if:
- You suffer from blurred vision and muscle weakness after eating contaminated food

 See also Nausea and vomiting, p.109; Diarrhoea, p.116.

 ## See your doctor first

Make an appointment to see your doctor if:

- You have severe abdominal pain or vomiting
- There is blood or mucus in your stools

What you can do yourself

You can treat a mild case of food poisoning at home using the following measures. You should feel better within a day or two.

- Get plenty of rest and make yourself as comfortable as possible.

- Drink at least 8 glasses of clear fluids a day. Take small sips so that you don't vomit. If necessary, take an oral rehydration preparation (*see* DRUG REMEDIES, right).

- As soon as you can eat, have bland foods such as boiled rice, pasta, and mashed potatoes. Start with small amounts, returning to your normal diet once you can eat these foods without problems. You should avoid tea, coffee, dairy products, alcohol, and fatty or spicy foods until a few days after the diarrhoea has stopped.

- Be careful about hygiene to avoid passing on the infection to other people. Wash your hands thoroughly after going to the toilet, and have your own towel. Don't make food for others, or share cutlery, cups, or plates. Keep away from those who are vulnerable to infections, such as young children, elderly people, and pregnant women.

- Take an antidiarrhoeal medicine if you need to stop diarrhoea quickly (*see* DRUG REMEDIES, right).

 DRUG REMEDIES

Oral rehydration preparations (*see* p.186) are designed to replace lost water, sugars, and salts. Make up a sachet with the recommended amount of water and drink the solution instead of or in addition to regular drinks.

Antidiarrhoeal drugs (*see* p.177) should be used only as a last resort because diarrhoea is the body's way of getting rid of infection. You can take loperamide for quick relief if diarrhoea is likely to cause embarrassment, for example, at work.

PREVENTION

Food hygiene Follow these steps to prevent germs from multiplying and avoid food poisoning.

- Before preparing food, wash your hands with warm water and soap, and dry them on a clean hand towel.
- Keep raw and ready-to-eat foods separate. Store raw meat in the bottom of the fridge so it can't drip down.
- Use different chopping boards and work surfaces for raw meat, cooked meat, and vegetables. Clean boards and surfaces thoroughly after use.
- Cook food thoroughly, especially meat, fish, or eggs.
- When reheating food, ensure that it is very hot all the way through. Don't reheat it more than once.

Seek further medical advice

Arrange to see your doctor if your symptoms are getting worse or have not cleared up within 28–48 hours.

Constipation

The normal frequency of bowel movements can vary from 3 times a day to 3 times a week, and most people have a regular habit. However, if you pass hard stools less than 3 times a week, you are probably constipated. Other symptoms include bloating, nausea, and cramping in your lower abdomen. Eating a diet that is low in fibre, not drinking enough fluids, having a sedentary lifestyle, and/or repeatedly ignoring the urge to go to the toilet can contribute to constipation. Some medicines, such as certain painkillers and iron supplements, may cause or aggravate the problem. Occasionally, constipation is caused by an underlying illness.

 ## See your doctor first

Arrange to see your doctor if you have unexplained changes in your bowel habit, or:

- You are passing blood, mucus, or pus
- You have severe pain in your abdomen
- You are losing weight

What you can do yourself

There are various ways to treat a mild bout of constipation and prevent it from recurring.

- Some foods, such as prunes and figs, have natural laxative properties, so include these with your meals. Don't skip breakfast. Having a hot drink with breakfast helps to stimulate the bowels.

- Drink at least 8 glasses of water and/or fruit juice a day. Cut down on tea, coffee, and cola, which can make you dehydrated.

- Try to do 20–30 minutes of exercise, such as walking, cycling, or swimming, every day, as activity helps to stimulate the bowels.

 - If other measures have not helped, try taking a fibre supplement (*see* NATURAL REMEDIES, right).

 - Use a stimulant laxative if constipation is severe or persistent (*see* DRUG REMEDIES, right).

 ## Seek further medical advice

Arrange to see your doctor if:

- Constipation has not cleared up after 7 days
- You have not had a normal bowel movement but have had leakage of faeces or diarrhoea
- You get recurrent bouts of constipation

 ### NATURAL REMEDIES

Fibre supplements (*see* LAXATIVES, p.185) make stools softer, bulkier, and easier to pass. The most common type is bran, which can be mixed with cereal, soup, or fruit juice. Start with a small amount and increase gradually. If bran is unpalatable, try a product containing ispaghula husk or methylcellulose.

 ### DRUG REMEDIES

Stimulant laxatives (*see* LAXATIVES, p.185), such as senna, can be used for temporary relief, but long-term or excessive use of stimulant laxatives may make you more constipated because your bowels no longer move efficiently without them.

 ### PREVENTION

Avoiding constipation The following measures will ensure that constipation doesn't recur.

- Go to the toilet when you have the urge; don't wait. Allow adequate time for bowel movements.
- Increase your fibre intake by gradually adding foods such as muesli, wholemeal bread, vegetables, and nuts to your diet. Drink plenty of fluids with the fibre.

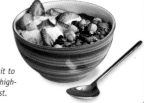

Healthy breakfast
Add fresh fruit to muesli for a high-fibre breakfast.

Diarrhoea

During an attack of diarrhoea, you pass loose or watery faeces frequently. You may also lose your appetite and have vomiting, abdominal cramps, bloating, and a headache. If the problem continues, you can become dehydrated due to the loss of large amounts of fluids and salts from your body. Diarrhoea is normally caused by bacteria or viruses found in infected food or transmitted from one person to another. In addition, some drugs, such as antibiotics, can cause short-term diarrhoea. An episode of diarrhoea normally clears up within a few days, but ongoing or recurrent diarrhoea can indicate an underlying bowel condition.

 See also Food intolerance, p.113; Food poisoning, p.114.

 ## See your doctor first

Make an appointment to see your doctor if:

- You have severe pain in your abdomen and/or you are vomiting
- You notice blood or mucus in your faeces

What you can do yourself

A mild episode of diarrhoea will clear up on its own in a few days. The following steps will ease symptoms and help prevent dehydration.

- Drink at least 8 glasses a day of clear liquids such as water and thin soups. If you are vomiting, have a drink beside you all the time and take frequent small sips. Passing small volumes of dark urine indicates that you are becoming dehydrated and need to drink more.

 - Try taking an oral rehydration preparation (*see* DRUG REMEDIES, right).

- Gradually start eating again as soon as you feel able. Start with bland foods such as boiled rice, pasta, mashed potatoes, and dry toast. Avoid tea, coffee, and cola, dairy products, alcohol, and fatty and spicy foods while you have diarrhoea and for a few days after it has cleared up.

 - It is best to let diarrhoea run its course because it is the body's way of eliminating infection. You can, however, use antidiarrhoeal drugs as a short-term solution when you are out, at work, or going on a long journey (*see* DRUG REMEDIES, right).

 - Take a painkiller if you have fever or headaches with the diarrhoea (*see* DRUG REMEDIES, right).

 ### DRUG REMEDIES

Oral rehydration preparations (*see* p.186) replace water, sugars, and salts lost from the body during an attack of diarrhoea. They are available as sachets of powder, to be made up with a recommended amount of drinking water. Drink the mixture instead of, or in addition to, regular drinks.

Antidiarrhoeal drugs (*see* p.177) such as loperamide work by slowing down bowel activity. Usually, 2 capsules are taken immediately, followed by 1 capsule after each loose stool. Don't take more than 8 capsules in 24 hours.

Painkillers Paracetamol (*see* p.187) will help reduce fever and discomfort and is less likely to irritate your bowels than other painkillers.

Oral rehydration
Stir the powder into the correct measure of water.

 ## Seek further medical advice

Arrange to see your doctor if:

- The diarrhoea gets worse
- There is no improvement in 24–48 hours

Piles

Piles (haemorrhoids) are swollen veins that develop in or around the anus. They mainly affect people who are constipated, who frequently strain when opening their bowels, or have repeated episodes of diarrhoea. The most common symptom is bright red blood on toilet paper or in the toilet bowl. Opening your bowels may be painful and it may feel as if they have not emptied completely. Sitting down may be uncomfortable. The skin around your anus may be itchy and irritated. Piles can also protrude outside the anus and form a painful swelling. The condition is more common in pregnant women and overweight people.

 See also Constipation, p.115; Diarrhoea, opposite page; Itchy anus, p.118.

See your doctor first

Make an appointment to see your doctor if:

- You have bleeding from your anus and/or a lump inside or near the anus

What you can do yourself

Piles can be uncomfortable, but there are several measures that you can take to help relieve them and support any treatment from your doctor.

- Treat constipation promptly to avoid triggering or aggravating piles. Small piles often subside once constipation is relieved.

- Go to the toilet as soon as you feel the need. Don't strain or hold your breath when opening your bowels, and don't rush. Even if it feels as if you have not emptied your bowels, resist the urge to strain at the end of a bowel movement.

- Clean your anal area after each bowel movement with a moist cloth or unscented, moist toilet tissue.

- If possible, sit in a shallow, warm bath for about 15 minutes, 3 or 4 times a day. Don't use soap to wash your anal area. Pat the area dry afterwards.

 - Take a painkiller to reduce the discomfort (*see* DRUG REMEDIES, right).

- If you have a painful, protruding pile, rest in bed for a day. Apply an ice pack (crushed ice in a bag or a bag of frozen vegetables, wrapped in a wet towel) to the anus for 15–20 minutes up to 4 times a day.

 - Try an over-the-counter haemorrhoid preparation (*see* DRUG REMEDIES, right).

DRUG REMEDIES

Painkillers Taking paracetamol (*see* p.187) or ibuprofen (*see* p.184) can help to relieve the discomfort of piles. If the pain persists for more than a few days, however, stop taking the painkillers and consult your doctor.

Haemorrhoid preparations (*see* p.182) are available as creams, ointments, and suppositories. They soothe painful piles and make it easier to open your bowels. Some contain a local anaesthetic to numb the area and help relieve irritation, or steroids to reduce inflammation. Don't use haemorrhoid preparations for longer than 6–7 days as you may develop a reaction to the ingredients, which may cause further irritation.

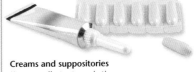

Creams and suppositories
Use an applicator to apply the cream; insert suppositories into the anus.

 ## Seek further medical advice

Arrange to see your doctor if:

- The bleeding gets worse
- Bleeding, irritation, or pain does not subside after a few days of treatment

Itchy anus

Anal itching is uncomfortable and may be embarrassing because you will have a strong urge to scratch. The skin around your anus may be red and sore, and may bleed and become infected if you scratch a great deal. Itching is often worse after emptying your bowels, and at night. In most cases, an itchy anus is due to irritation from toiletries, or from sweat, moisture, or traces of faeces left in contact with the skin. People who are overweight, sweat profusely, and/or wear tight-fitting underwear are more susceptible. Sometimes a particular food contributes to the problem. Piles and threadworms are common causes of itching.

 See also Piles, p.117; Threadworms, p.137.

See your doctor first

Make an appointment to see your doctor if:

- You have anal bleeding or a mucus discharge
- You have pain and/or a lump near your anus

What you can do yourself

Anal itching can usually be relieved with home treatment, which may also help prevent recurrences.

- Resist the urge to scratch. Cut your fingernails short and wear cotton gloves at night.

 - Try a sedative antihistamine to reduce itching and help you sleep (*see* DRUG REMEDIES, right).

- Wash your anus morning and evening with plain water and pat the area dry. Make sure the area is completely dry – using a hairdryer may be helpful.

- Applying a haemorrhoid cream after washing may soothe itching (*see* DRUG REMEDIES, right). Alternatively, use calendula cream (*see* NATURAL REMEDIES, right). Place a thin strip of cotton wool or tissue next to your anus to absorb moisture.

- Wash after each bowel movement. When this is not possible, use a moistened cloth or unscented, moist toilet tissues. Use plain toilet tissue after passing urine to dry yourself thoroughly.

- Wear loose cotton underwear, and change it daily or more often if necessary. Avoid wearing tight-fitting trousers or tights.

- Try to identify and then cut down on food or drink that may be contributing to anal itching, such as beer, coffee, tomatoes, or spicy foods.

DRUG REMEDIES

Antihistamines (*see* p.178) relieve itching. Taking a sedative antihistamine, available as tablets or syrup, will also help you to sleep.

Haemorrhoid preparations (*see* p.182) contain ingredients such as zinc oxide that help to soothe the area around the anus. Don't use them for longer than 6–7 days because you may develop a reaction that causes further irritation.

NATURAL REMEDIES

Calendula cream (*see* p.179) is a mild, soothing cream made from extracts of the calendula (marigold) plant. Apply it once a day after washing. Discontinue if you develop a reaction to the cream.

Using calendula
Apply calendula cream sparingly and rub it in lightly.

Seek further medical advice

Arrange to see your doctor if:

- The itchiness does not subside after about a week of using the above measures
- You develop any new symptoms or other family members develop an itch

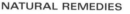

MEN'S PROBLEMS

Painful scrotum

Minor injury to the scrotum does not usually cause lasting harm, but sudden severe pain can be due to torsion (twisting) of one of the testicles inside, which can cause permanent damage. A painful, tender scrotum, sometimes with swelling, may be due to an infection (epididymitis). You may also have a fever and pain passing urine. Other causes of pain include mumps and, rarely, testicular cancer.

> ## WARNING
>
> Seek immediate medical help if:
> - You develop sudden or severe pain in the scrotum
> - Pain after an injury to the area persists for more than an hour

See also Mumps, p.26.

 ## See your doctor first

Arrange to see your doctor promptly if:

- You have had mild pain for more than 2 days
- You think you have epididymitis
- You find a lump in the scrotum or testes

What you can do yourself

Try the following home treatments alone or in conjunction with treatment from your doctor.

- To relieve pain and swelling, apply an ice pack (such as a bag of frozen peas or crushed ice in a plastic bag wrapped in a wet towel) to the testicles. Hold for about 10 minutes. Use twice a day. You can also take a painkiller (*see* DRUG REMEDIES, right).

- Lie on your back with a rolled-up towel placed between your legs and under the scrotum to lift it and relieve discomfort. When moving around, wear an athletic support or two pairs of close-fitting underpants, especially if the testicles are swollen.

- When the pain has eased, check your testicles regularly for lumps (*see* PRACTICAL TECHNIQUE, right).

 ## Seek further medical advice

Arrange to see your doctor if:

- The pain is worse or no better after 2 days

DRUG REMEDIES

Painkillers can be used to reduce pain and swelling in the scrotum and also fever. Take an anti-inflammatory painkiller such as ibuprofen (*see* p.184).

PRACTICAL TECHNIQUE

Testicular self-examination All men should examine their testicles regularly to detect lumps or other changes that may be an early sign of cancer.

- Examine yourself once a month after a warm bath, when the scrotum is relaxed. Check for any lumps or swellings. Both testicles should be smooth except along the top and back, where you will feel a soft tube (epididymis) that carries and stores sperm.
- It is common for one testicle to be slightly larger and/or hang lower than the other but any noticeable increase in size or weight may indicate a problem. If you notice any changes in either your testicles or scrotum, consult your doctor promptly.

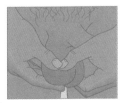

Examining your testicles
Carefully roll your fingers and thumb across the entire surface of each testicle in turn.

Painful penis

The skin on the penis is thin and delicate and is easily injured or irritated. Minor bruising and chafing may occur after playing sports or sexual activity. Soreness at the tip may be due to poor hygiene or irritation from soaps or spermicides, or result from infections, including sexually transmitted infections (STIs). Other symptoms of an STI include a rash, discharge from the penis, and pain when passing urine. Pain that occurs only when your penis is erect or during sex may be due to an overtight foreskin.

> **WARNING**
>
> Seek immediate medical help if:
> - You have a painful erection that lasts long after arousal has passed
> - You have difficulty rolling your foreskin forwards again after it has been retracted

⊕ See your doctor first

Arrange to see your doctor, or go to a genito-urinary medicine (GUM) clinic if:

- You suspect that you have a sexually transmitted infection or you are not sure what is causing the pain

What you can do yourself

There are several measures you can take that will ease pain and help prevent soreness.

- Keep your penis and foreskin clean. Have a bath or shower every day. If you have a foreskin, wash underneath it with water and unperfumed soap. Dry the end of your penis thoroughly.

- Wear loose underwear to avoid discomfort.

- If the head of your penis gets inflamed or sore during sex, apply a water-soluble lubricating jelly beforehand (see DRUG REMEDIES, right). Wash your genitals after intercourse. If you think the problem is due to the condoms you use, switch to a non-allergenic type or one with a different spermicide.

- If you have a small injury on the tip of your penis, let it heal completely before having sex again.

- If you think you may be sensitive to soaps and washing powders, use only non-biological powder for your underclothes and avoid fabric softeners.

- If you have a sexually transmitted infection, bathing with salt water will help relieve symptoms (see PRACTICAL TIP, right). Tell your partner you have an STI; he or she may also need treatment.

DRUG REMEDIES

Lubricating jelly (see p.185) is widely available and will make sex more comfortable. Use it to help prevent soreness that may develop because of irritants or vigorous activity.

Using jelly
Apply a water-soluble lubricant to your penis just before intercourse.

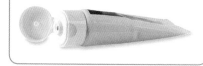

PRACTICAL TIP

Salt-water baths Gently bathing your penis 2 or 3 times a day in warm, salty water will help relieve soreness, swelling, and inflammation. Add a handful of salt to a bath two-thirds full. If you are finding urination uncomfortable or painful, pass urine while lying in a warm bath, and shower yourself and the bath afterwards.

⊕ Seek further medical advice

Arrange to see your doctor or go to a genito-urinary medicine (GUM) clinic if:

- Pain in your penis persists, or you develop new symptoms

Urinary problems in men

Many urinary problems in men that start in later life are due to enlargement of the prostate gland, which lies beneath the bladder. This condition is usually noncancerous (in which case it is called benign prostatic hyperplasia), but sometimes it is due to cancer. The prostate may constrict the bladder outlet, causing symptoms such as an urgent or frequent need to pass urine (including at night); a weak flow; dribbling afterwards; and a feeling that your bladder has not emptied completely.

WARNING

Seek immediate medical help if:
- You develop pain or swelling in your abdomen and can't pass urine

✚ See your doctor first

Make an appointment to see your doctor if:

- You have problems when passing urine, especially if there is blood in the urine or you feel a burning sensation
- You are taking an over-the-counter or prescribed medicine that may be making the problem worse, such as a decongestant or an antidepressant

What you can do yourself

Use these self-help measures alongside treatment from your doctor to help minimize urinary problems.

- Drink 6–8 glasses of fluid a day so your urine doesn't get too concentrated and cause irritation. Avoid drinking too much over a short time, however, as this may cause a sudden urge to pass urine.

- Pass urine only when your bladder feels full. Take your time so that your bladder empties completely. Sometimes sitting on the toilet is more effective.

- If you often need to get up at night, drink less in the evening and stop drinking a few hours before bedtime. Empty your bladder before going to bed.

- Reduce your intake of tea, coffee, cola, and alcohol. These drinks make your bladder fill quickly and cause a sudden or urgent need to pass urine.

- Avoid carbonated drinks, citrus fruits and juices, and spicy foods, as they may irritate your bladder.

- Try saw palmetto if you have noncancerous prostate enlargement (see NATURAL REMEDIES, right).

NATURAL REMEDIES

Saw palmetto (see p.188) preparations are made from the berries of the saw palmetto plant. You can take them to improve urine flow and bladder emptying if you have noncancerous prostate enlargement. However, if you have symptoms of prostate enlargement, you should always talk to your doctor before taking saw palmetto.

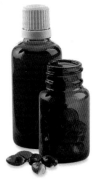

Taking saw palmetto
You may have to take saw palmetto tincture, capsules, or tablets for 1–3 months before you see an improvement in your urinary symptoms.

✋ PREVENTION

Reducing urinary problems The following lifestyle changes and remedies may lead to a long-term improvement in urinary symptoms.

- Excess weight puts pressure on your bladder, so try to lose some weight if you need to do so.
- Taking regular exercise can help to reduce symptoms caused by an enlarged prostate, while a sedentary lifestyle tends to make them worse.

Erectile dysfunction (impotence)

Most men experience occasional difficulty in getting or maintaining an erection, often because of stress, tiredness, drinking too much alcohol, or a recent illness. Temporary erectile dysfunction is unlikely to be a cause for concern if you are still able to achieve an erection by masturbating or if you sometimes wake with an erection. Long-term erectile dysfunction can be due to illnesses, such as circulatory diseases and diabetes, or drugs, such as diuretics and antidepressants. It may also be caused by anxiety or depression, or relationship problems. As you get older, it may take longer to get an erection and it may be less firm.

 ## See your doctor first

Make an appointment to see your doctor if:

● You suffer regularly from erectile dysfunction or if you are taking a prescribed drug that may be causing the problem

What you can do yourself

There are several things you can do that may help you overcome temporary erectile dysfunction.

● Don't judge yourself harshly. If you are stressed or tired, for example, because of money worries, work, or recent illness, tackle the underlying problem.

 ●If you are in a long-term relationship, talk to your partner. Share your worries, and work together in order to try to solve the problem. It may help if there is less pressure on you to "perform", so if erectile dysfunction is making you nervous about sexual intercourse, try ways of sharing intimacy that reduce sexual anxiety (*see* PRACTICAL TECHNIQUE, right).

● To help relieve anxiety, try practising deep breathing and muscle relaxation exercises (*see* PRACTICAL TECHNIQUES, pp.20–21).

● Reduce your alcohol intake; even better, avoid it altogether. Drinking too much alcohol can cause difficulty in getting an erection; recreational drugs can have a similar effect.

● Stop smoking, or at least cut down if you smoke heavily. Young men who smoke double their risk of long-term erectile dysfunction in later life.

 ### PRACTICAL TECHNIQUE

Reducing sexual anxiety Worrying about getting an erection can set up a cycle of "performance anxiety". One of the best ways to reduce anxiety is to take things slowly.

● Take the pressure off. Take turns to explore your partner's body using stroking and massage. You should agree there will be no touching of genitals or breasts at this stage. This will help you both relax.
● After several of these sessions, allow genital and breast stimulation, too, but refrain from intercourse.
● Continue relaxed and leisurely stroking and massage until you begin to get erections again and feel comfortable about proceeding to intercourse.

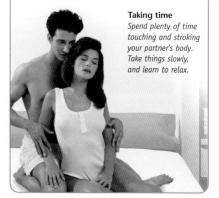

Taking time
Spend plenty of time touching and stroking your partner's body. Take things slowly, and learn to relax.

 ## Seek further medical advice

Arrange to see your doctor if:

●The measures above do not help or if you think erectile dysfunction may have a physical cause

Premature ejaculation

Premature ejaculation is a common sexual problem, especially for young men, in which a man reaches orgasm and ejaculates with minimum stimulation, just before or shortly after penetration. The problem is mainly due to excitement and/or anxiety and often occurs at the start of a new relationship and resolves itself over time. However, recurrent premature ejaculation can be physically and emotionally frustrating for both partners and may harm a relationship. Stress and depression aggravate the condition; some men become so anxious they develop erectile dysfunction. Rarely, the cause is a prostate or nervous system problem.

 See also Erectile dysfunction (impotence), opposite page.

What you can do yourself

Because anxiety is a major part of premature ejaculation, talking about the problem with your partner may help to resolve it. There are also several techniques you can try.

● If you are in a long-term relationship, share your feelings with your partner. Discuss the problem calmly and good-humouredly when you are not engaged in sex. Don't blame yourself or feel guilty.

● Some men find wearing a condom dulls sensation sufficiently to delay ejaculation. Some types of condom have a desensitizing lubricant inside that contains a mild topical anaesthetic. These may be even more effective. Don't try using anaesthetic gel without a condom – it will reduce sensation in your partner, too.

 ● Try using the squeeze technique (*see* PRACTICAL TECHNIQUE, right) to help you control ejaculation.

● Focus your attention on your partner's pleasure during foreplay and delay penetration for as long as possible. If your partner is close to or has reached orgasm before penetration, you will both feel less anxious about premature ejaculation.

● During intercourse, distract yourself by thinking about something totally unrelated and rather dull: count backwards in threes or think about work.

● Try experimenting with different sexual positions. Having your partner on top, for example, may be less stimulating and help you delay ejaculation.

PRACTICAL TECHNIQUE

The squeeze technique This method of preventing premature ejaculation can be carried out by you or your partner.

● When you feel you're about to ejaculate, use your thumb and forefinger to squeeze the shaft of the penis just below the head, as shown below. This causes your erection to be partially lost, temporarily preventing ejaculation.
● By practising this technique regularly, you can achieve greater control over ejaculation, and this will boost your sexual confidence. Eventually, you will no longer need to use the technique.

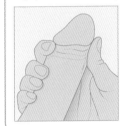

Apply pressure
Use the thumb and forefinger to apply pressure just behind the head of the penis, on the upper and lower sides.

⊕ Seek medical advice

Arrange to see your doctor if:

● You continue to experience premature ejaculation after following the advice here

WOMEN'S PROBLEMS

Breast pain and lumpy breasts

Many healthy women experience breast pain (mastalgia) or lumpiness. The symptoms normally affect both breasts and are usually related to hormonal changes during the menstrual cycle. A few days before your period your breasts may feel swollen, painful, tender, and/or lumpy. These symptoms usually go when the period is over. A more general tendency to breast lumpiness sometimes occurs during adolescence, during pregnancy, or when taking the contraceptive pill or hormone replacement therapy (HRT). Women who are breastfeeding sometimes develop a red, hot, painful area on one breast due to a build-up of milk or infection (mastitis). Although the majority of breast lumps are not cancer, persistent lumps should always be investigated.

 See also Premenstrual syndrome, p.127.

 ## See your doctor first

Arrange to see your doctor promptly if:

- You find a lump in your breast
- You have lumpiness that persists throughout your menstrual cycle
- You have persistent breast pain that is unrelated to periods, or pain in your armpit
- You think your symptoms may be due to taking the contraceptive pill or HRT
- You have symptoms of mastitis

What you can do yourself

Use the following measures to identify and to help alleviate cyclical breast pain or breast lumpiness. (For an attack of mastitis, follow the specific advice on the opposite page.)

- Keep a diary for 2 or 3 menstrual cycles, noting when your breasts become lumpy or sore and when the symptoms pass. This will help you to decide if the problem is related to your menstrual cycle.

- Make sure that all your bras fit properly. Try wearing a larger size in the week before your period, and/or wear a support bra, such as a sports bra, to reduce breast movement. You may find that wearing a soft bra at night also helps to make you feel more comfortable.

 ### DRUG REMEDIES

Painkillers, such as paracetamol (*see* p.187) or ibuprofen (*see* p.184) will help relieve discomfort for the few days each month when your breasts are painful. If you are breastfeeding, consult your doctor before you take any medication.

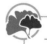 ### NATURAL REMEDIES

Vitamin B$_6$ supplements (*see* p.189) may help reduce or prevent cyclical breast pain or lumpiness. Usually, you will need to take the supplement for 2–3 months to feel any benefit. Don't exceed the recommended dose, because high doses can be harmful. To boost your intake of B$_6$ from your diet, eat foods such as poultry, eggs, soya, oats, wholegrain bread and cereal, bananas, and nuts.

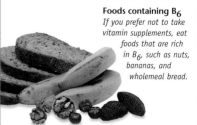

Foods containing B$_6$
If you prefer not to take vitamin supplements, eat foods that are rich in B$_6$, such as nuts, bananas, and wholemeal bread.

What you can do yourself *continued...*

- Reduce your caffeine intake by cutting down on drinks such as coffee, tea, and cola.

- If you suffer from fluid retention and bloating, cut down on salt in the week before your period.

- Increase the amount of carbohydrates in your diet, eat plenty of fresh fruit and vegetables, and avoid fatty food.

- If you are overweight, try losing some weight. Excess fat stores in your body can affect your hormone levels and contribute to breast pain.

- If tension or stress makes you more susceptible to cyclical breast pain, try practising some deep breathing and muscle relaxation exercises (*see* PRACTICAL TECHNIQUES, pp.20–21).

 - Take a painkiller on the days when your breasts are painful (*see* DRUG REMEDIES, left).

 - Some women find supplements of vitamin B_6 help to ease cyclical breast pain and lumpiness (*see* NATURAL REMEDIES, opposite page).

 - Regularly examine your breasts for lumps (*see* PRACTICAL TECHNIQUE, right).

Mastitis

- Make sure your baby is latched on correctly and is sucking properly (*see* PRACTICAL TIPS: BREASTFEEDING HOLDS FOR SORE NIPPLES, p.126). This will help relieve pressure on the breast and may also help prevent mastitis.

- If you are breastfeeding and you have pain in one breast due to mastitis or milk build-up (engorgement), continue to feed your baby regularly from the affected breast, unless your doctor has advised you otherwise. This will keep the milk flowing and stop the breast getting too full. Alternatively, use a breast pump.

Seek further medical advice

Arrange to see your doctor if:

- Cyclical breast pain or lumpiness has lasted for more than 2–3 menstrual cycles and is not relieved using self-help measures
- Breast pain is causing you distress and/or is preventing you from carrying out your normal daily activities

PRACTICAL TECHNIQUE

Breast awareness If you are familiar with the normal appearance and feel of your breasts at different times it will enable you to recognize if any abnormal changes occur. Every woman's breasts are unique so what is normal for one woman may not be for another. It is therefore important for every woman to know what is normal for her personally. In addition, a woman's breasts vary in appearance and feel depending on her age and the stage of her menstrual cycle (if she has not undergone the menopause).

However, there are general differences in the breasts at different times of life. Before the menopause, the breasts tend to feel different at different times during the menstrual cycle. In the days preceding a period, the milk-producing glands become active and the breasts may feel lumpy and tender. After the menopause, the milk-producing glands are no longer active and the breasts tend to be less firm, softer, and not lumpy. In women who have had a hysterectomy (removal of the uterus), the breasts usually show the regular monthly changes until the time at which the menopause would otherwise have occurred.

There are many possible causes for changes in the breasts, and most are not serious. However any changes need to be checked by a doctor without delay because there is a small chance they could be an early sign of cancer. The following are the changes you should be aware of:

- Any lumps or thickened areas of tissue in one breast or armpit that are different from the corresponding part of the other breast or armpit.
- Any alterations in either the shape or outline of your breasts, particularly any changes that occur when you move your arms or when your breasts lift.
- Any dimpling or puckering of the skin of your breasts.
- Any pain or discomfort in one breast that is different from usual.
- Any rash on or around your nipples, or any bleeding or moist areas on your nipples that do not heal readily.
- Any change in the position of your nipples.
- Any discharge from your nipples (unless you are breastfeeding and it is a milky discharge).

Cracked nipples

Many new mothers develop sore, tender nipples during the first few weeks of breastfeeding. One or both nipples may be painful, red, and ridged and may bleed if the skin cracks. Cracked nipples tend to occur when a baby is not positioned properly at the breast and sucks only on the end of the nipple. Women with flat or inverted nipples are susceptible. Sometimes, cracked nipples are due to the fungal infection thrush.

 See also Feeding problems, pp.144–145.

 ## See your doctor first

Arrange to see your doctor promptly if:

- Your nipples are red and shiny and have a white deposit on them
- There is a red, tender area on your breast

What you can do yourself

Cracked nipples usually heal quickly once you and your baby develop a good breastfeeding technique.

- Check the way you hold your baby at the breast (*see* PRACTICAL TECHNIQUE: SUCCESSFUL BREASTFEEDING, p.144). Using a new hold may help to reduce pain (*see* PRACTICAL TIPS, right).

- Feed your baby on demand and offer the nipple that is least sore first, when your baby is sucking hardest. Breathe deeply as your baby latches on: a sore nipple is most painful for the first few sucks.

- For flat or inverted nipples, use a lightweight plastic nipple shield to help pull out your nipples.

- Try using a lanolin cream to help heal deep, painful cracks (*see* DRUG REMEDIES, right).

- After each feed, wash your nipples with warm water and dry them carefully. Don't use plastic-backed breast pads; they trap moisture. Expose your breasts to the air whenever you can.

- If your nipples are very painful, take paracetamol (*see* DRUG REMEDIES, right).

 ## Seek further medical advice

Consult your doctor or breastfeeding advisor if:

- Your nipples are not healing within 2–3 days

PRACTICAL TIPS

Breastfeeding holds for sore nipples Holding your baby higher and well supported will reduce painful tugging on a sore nipple.

- Cradle your baby's head high in the crook of the arm with the tummy against your own and the mouth directly facing your nipple. Tuck your baby's arm around your body and keep the bottom well supported. Make sure your baby takes the nipple and the darker area around it (areola) into the mouth.
- As an occasional alternative, try the football hold to even out sucking on sore nipples. Using a pillow for support, tuck your baby under your arm with the feet towards your back (like an American football).

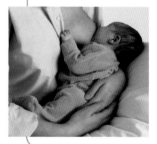

Maintaining good support *Hold your baby with his or her front against your body, and support him or her securely.*

DRUG REMEDIES

Lanolin ointment (*see* p.184) formulated for breastfeeding mothers will soothe sore nipples. Rub in a little to protect the skin and help cracks to heal. You don't need to wipe it off before feeds.

Paracetamol (*see* p.187) will reduce discomfort and so help you relax while your baby feeds. Take a dose 30 minutes before a feed.

Premenstrual syndrome (PMS)

Women with premenstrual syndrome (PMS) are troubled by a variety of symptoms that start about 7 days before a menstrual period and ease when the period begins. You may feel irritable, angry, depressed, or anxious for no particular reason. You may also be absentminded and find it hard to concentrate. Physical symptoms include headache, sleep problems, food cravings, constipation, bloating, weight gain, and breast tenderness or lumpiness. Hormone imbalances and stress contribute to the problem.

 See also Difficulty sleeping, p.17; Poor memory, p.25; Headache, p.85; Bloating and flatulence, p.108; Constipation, p.115; Breast pain and lumpy breasts, pp.124–125.

See your doctor first

Arrange to see your doctor if you are not sure that your symptoms are due to PMS.

What you can do yourself

There are a number of remedies that may help PMS. Use them before the first symptoms develop.

● Eat regularly to keep your sugar levels steady and prevent you becoming nervy and irritable. Have plenty of carbohydrates, such as pasta and potatoes, and increase your intake of fruit and vegetables. Avoid sugary snacks; if you are hungry between meals, eat fruit or a wholemeal biscuit.

● Reduce your intake of salt; use herbs and spices to flavour your food instead.

● Drink 6–8 glasses of water a day, and cut down on caffeinated drinks such as coffee. Avoid alcohol in the days before your period.

● Use memory aids such as a jotter or message board to keep track of things you need to do.

● Try to reduce stress (*see* pp.20–21). Postpone big plans and changes, and avoid difficult decisions.

● Go out in the fresh air if possible and take a brisk walk. Get plenty of sleep at night.

Seek further medical advice

Arrange to see your doctor if:

● You still have PMS symptoms after following this advice, or symptoms become worse

PREVENTION

Controlling PMS These longer-term steps may prevent some symptoms of PMS developing and help you cope better with those that remain.

● Keep a diary for 3 months, noting any factors that make PMS symptoms worse, such as particular foods or stress at work, so you can avoid them in future.

● Try a course of vitamin B$_6$ to help prevent symptoms (*see* NATURAL REMEDIES, below).

● Go for a brisk walk for 20–30 minutes, 5 days a week, or try swimming or practising yoga regularly.

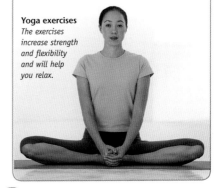

Yoga exercises
The exercises increase strength and flexibility and will help you relax.

NATURAL REMEDIES

Vitamin B$_6$ There is evidence that vitamin B$_6$ (*see* p.189) helps prevent PMS. You may need to take a supplement for 2–3 months before you feel any benefit. Alternatively, boost your diet with foods rich in B$_6$, such as chicken, eggs, bananas, and nuts.

Painful periods

Many women have a cramping pain in their lower abdomen just before, or at the start of, their monthly period. Some women also have headaches, backache, nausea, and diarrhoea. Stress and tension can make symptoms worse. Painful periods most commonly affect younger women and often become less severe with age or after childbirth. They don't usually have a serious underlying cause.

> **WARNING**
>
> Seek immediate medical help if:
> ● You have lower abdominal pain and vaginal bleeding and there is a risk that you might be pregnant

➡ *See also* Diarrhoea, p.116; Premenstrual syndrome (PMS), p.127.

What you can do yourself

You can usually relieve the symptoms of painful periods using self-help measures.

● To relieve abdominal pain and other aches and pains, take ibuprofen (*see* DRUG REMEDIES, right). You can also soak in a warm bath or apply heat to your abdomen using a hot-water bottle wrapped in a towel or a heating pad.

● Taking exercise, such as a brisk walk, may bring relief because it stimulates muscles to produce natural painkilling chemicals called endorphins. In the longer term, regular exercise may also help to prevent painful periods or reduce their severity.

● Try to avoid stress and tasks that you find physically and/or mentally tiring.

● To reduce anxiety and tension, try practising some deep breathing and muscle relaxation exercises (*see* PRACTICAL TECHNIQUES, pp.20–21).

● Taking vitamin B₆ supplements and/or eating oily fish containing essential fatty acids may help to reduce period pain (*see* NATURAL REMEDIES, right).

⊕ Seek medical advice

Arrange to see your doctor if:

● You have bleeding between periods
● Pains continue after your period has finished and/or you have an offensive vaginal discharge
● You wish to discuss taking the contraceptive pill, which may help to reduce period pains
● The measures given above are not helping to control the pain

DRUG REMEDIES

Ibuprofen (*see* p.184) is an anti-inflammatory drug that helps to reduce cramping and bleeding. If you are prone to period pains, begin taking it before you expect your period to start. If you can't take ibuprofen, you can use paracetamol (*see* p.187).

NATURAL REMEDIES

Vitamin B₆ supplements (*see* p.189) may help relieve symptoms. Alternatively, eat foods that are rich in the vitamin, such as nuts, soya, and bananas.

Oily fish such as salmon and mackerel contain omega-3 essential fatty acids (*see* p.181), which are thought to affect levels of prostaglandin, a hormone that causes period pains.

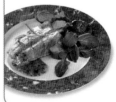

Omega-3 source
Try to include oily fish, such as salmon, in your diet about 2–3 times a week.

PREVENTION

Stopping smoking You may be able to prevent or reduce period pain by giving up smoking. This is because smoking has been shown to increase the strength and duration of menstrual cramps.

Menopausal problems

The menopause is a natural change that usually occurs in women between 45 and 55 years, due to falling levels of the female hormone oestrogen. At first, your periods become irregular and scanty; then they stop. You are considered to be menopausal when you haven't had a period for a year. Some women have no further symptoms, but others have various problems, including hot flushes, night sweats, vaginal dryness, dry skin, urinary problems, thinning bones, irritability, depression, and poor concentration or memory.

 See also Feeling depressed, pp.22–23; Poor memory, p.25; Dry skin, p.41; Poor bladder control, p.131; Painful intercourse, p.134.

See your doctor first

Make an appointment to see your doctor if you are unsure whether your symptoms are due to the menopause, or if you wish to discuss hormone replacement therapy.

What you can do yourself

A few self-help measures may be all you need to control menopausal symptoms.

- If you get hot flushes, dress in layers that you can easily remove. Sleep in a cool room under a light duvet or blanket. Have showers, or warm rather than hot baths. Avoid spicy and hot foods, and cut down on coffee, tea, and alcohol.

- If you have vaginal dryness and find sex painful, try a lubricating jelly (*see* DRUG REMEDIES, right).

- Eat calcium-rich foods to help prevent bone thinning (*see* NATURAL REMEDIES, right). Go out in the sun from time to time; sunlight stimulates vitamin D production, which helps your body to absorb calcium.

- Try including soya products, which contain phyto-oestrogens, in your diet (*see* NATURAL REMEDIES, right).

- Drink lots of water: 6–8 glasses a day.

- If you're feeling tense, try practising muscle relaxation exercises (*see* PRACTICAL TECHNIQUE, p.21).

- Take regular weight-bearing exercise to relieve stress and strengthen your bones. Brisk walking for about 20–30 minutes a day, 5 days a week, is ideal.

- Avoid smoking – it can worsen symptoms and increase the risk of heart disease and stroke.

DRUG REMEDIES

Lubricating jelly (*see* p.185) will help to make sexual intercourse more comfortable. You can either use a gel just before intercourse to lubricate the vagina, or try a longer-acting vaginal moisturizer.

NATURAL REMEDIES

Calcium is found in many foods, including dark green, leafy vegetables such as broccoli; dairy products; tinned fish with edible bones, such as sardines or salmon; nuts; and bread.

Phyto-oestrogens (*see* p.187) are natural plant chemicals, found in soya-based foods, that act like oestrogen in the body. Eating foods rich in phyto-oestrogens, such as soya beans, tofu, and soya milk, may help reduce hot flushes and strengthen bones.

Stir-fried tofu
Rich in phyto-oestrogens, tofu can be included in many healthy meals.

Seek further medical advice

Arrange to see your doctor if:

- Self-help is not relieving your symptoms
- You develop new symptoms, such as vaginal bleeding, after having had no periods for 1 year

Cystitis

Cystitis is inflammation of the bladder, usually as a result of an infection in the urine. If you have an attack of cystitis, you will probably feel a burning pain when you pass urine and have the urge to pass urine frequently, even when your bladder is empty. The urine may be cloudy and foul-smelling, and you may have pain in your lower abdomen. Attacks are sometimes triggered by sexual intercourse. Cystitis is a common condition in women, but is much less common in men and children.

 ## See your doctor first

Make an appointment to see your doctor if:

- You are pregnant
- There is blood in your urine
- You have pain in your back, or in your sides just below your ribs; high fever; or shivering
- Your symptoms are not relieved within 48 hours using the measures below

Men and children with symptoms of cystitis should always see a doctor.

What you can do yourself

Using these simple measures promptly may be enough to clear up a mild attack of cystitis.

- Drink plenty of fluids to wash away bacteria and keep the urine dilute. This will help make your urine less irritating to the bladder.

- Avoid citrus fruits, tomatoes, spicy foods, caffeine, alcohol, and nicotine. All of these substances can irritate the bladder.

- Try to pass urine immediately before and after sexual intercourse, to help flush out any bacteria.

 - Take cystitis relief preparations (*see* DRUG REMEDIES, right) to make your urine less acidic. Alternatively, make your own by dissolving a teaspoonful of sodium bicarbonate in a glass of water and drinking it 2 or 3 times a day.

 - Hold a covered hot-water bottle over your lower abdomen to relieve any pain, and/or take a painkiller (*see* DRUG REMEDIES, right).

 - Cranberry juice may help to relieve symptoms or even prevent cystitis (*see* NATURAL REMEDIES, right).

 ### DRUG REMEDIES

Cystitis relief preparations (*see* p.180) usually contain chemical compounds called citrates that make urine less acidic and relieve burning and irritation. They are available as granules, which you dissolve in water and drink.

Painkillers, such as paracetamol (*see* p.187), can help relieve some of the discomfort of cystitis.

 ### NATURAL REMEDIES

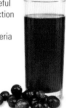 **Cranberry juice** is a useful treatment that helps to fight infection and may prevent recurrences of cystitis by reducing levels of bacteria in the bladder.

Drinking cranberry juice
Choose a juice with a high proportion of cranberry, and drink 1–2 glasses a day.

PREVENTION

Avoiding recurrences The following measures can help to prevent attacks of cystitis.

- Drink 8 glasses (2–3 litres) of fluids each day, including 1–2 glasses of cranberry juice.
- Empty your bladder frequently and completely.
- After a bowel movement, wipe from front to back to prevent bacteria from entering the urethra (the passage from the bladder to the outside of the body).
- Wear cotton underwear and avoid tight trousers.
- Don't use vaginal deodorants.
- Take showers instead of baths, if possible.

Poor bladder control

Many women suffer from poor bladder control. If you have a condition called stress incontinence, for example, you may leak small amounts of urine when you cough, sneeze, exercise, or lift something heavy. This can be due to weakness in the pelvic floor muscles (which support your bladder, womb, and rectum) and is common in women who have had children. Other causes of stress incontinence include constipation, urine infections, hormonal changes after the menopause, and some drugs (such as diuretics). Some women have a problem called urge incontinence, which causes sudden urges to pass urine or a large leakage without warning. This condition is sometimes due to a disorder that affects the nerves controlling the bladder.

 See also Constipation, p.115; **Cystitis,** opposite page.

See your doctor first

Make an appointment to see your doctor if:

- You have large leakages of urine
- You are also thirsty and drinking lots of fluid
- You leak urine without warning, or can't get to the toilet fast enough
- You are taking a prescribed medicine that may be causing poor bladder control

What you can do yourself

There are several steps you can take to improve bladder control if you have stress incontinence, or to supplement treatment from your doctor.

- Drink 6–8 glasses of fluid a day so that your urine doesn't become too concentrated, but don't drink too much in a short time as this may cause leaks.

- Get into the habit of passing urine only when your bladder feels full. Take your time on the toilet so that your bladder empties completely. Empty your bladder before going to bed at night.

- Cut down on tea, coffee, cola, and alcohol; they may cause a sudden and/or uncontrollable urge to pass urine. Avoid fizzy drinks, citrus fruits and juices, and spicy foods, as they may irritate your bladder.

 ● Do pelvic floor exercises every day (*see* PRACTICAL TECHNIQUE, right).

● If you leak urine during activities such as running or aerobics, insert a tampon just beforehand to help support the bladder. Remove it promptly afterwards. Use only as an occasional measure.

PRACTICAL TECHNIQUE

Pelvic floor exercises can be done anywhere, sitting or standing. It may take up to 12 weeks for you to benefit, and you will need to keep doing them to prevent symptoms from recurring.

- Tighten and release your pelvic floor muscles: these are the muscles you use to stop urinating mid-stream.
- Squeeze the muscles, hold for a few seconds, then relax slowly. Repeat several times. Gradually build up to 10 squeezes, taking 10 seconds for each and resting for about 4 seconds between squeezes.
- Do the exercises regularly throughout every day until they become second nature.

PREVENTION

Bladder care Over time, these measures will reduce pressure and irritation affecting your bladder.

- Try to lose any excess weight.
- Eat plenty of fibre to prevent constipation.
- Stop smoking. Nicotine irritates the bladder, and smoke can make you cough and strain your muscles.

Seek further medical advice

Arrange to see your doctor if:

- Incontinence gets worse
- You see little or no improvement in your bladder control after 4–6 weeks
- You develop other symptoms

Vaginal discharge

It is normal for a woman to have some discharge from the vagina. This is usually clear or white, the amount and consistency varying at different times in the menstrual cycle, during pregnancy, and in response to sexual arousal. However, a profuse discharge or one that has an unusual consistency or smell is usually a sign of infection. The most common cause is thrush, a yeast infection that produces a discharge like cottage cheese, irritation in or around your vagina and, sometimes, a burning sensation when you pass urine. Thrush is not usually sexually transmitted. It is caused by factors that encourage overgrowth of yeast, such as taking antibiotics, wearing tight-fitting clothes, and using vaginal douches and deodorants. Some types of vaginal discharge are a symptom of a sexually transmitted infection and need treatment from a doctor.

 ## See your doctor first

Make an appointment to see your doctor if you think you may have a sexually transmitted infection and/or:

- The discharge is bloodstained, greenish-yellow, or foul-smelling
- You have other symptoms, such as fever and lower abdominal pain
- You have recurrent abnormal discharges
- You are pregnant

What you can do yourself

If you are sure that you have thrush, you can usually treat it yourself. Start the treatment as soon as you notice symptoms.

 - Use an antifungal pessary, cream, tablet, or combination product for thrush (see DRUG REMEDIES, right).

 - To relieve itchiness and discomfort, add some sodium bicarbonate to a bath (see NATURAL REMEDIES, right).

 - For mild thrush, applying live yoghurt to your vulva and vagina may help (see NATURAL REMEDIES, right). This has a soothing effect.

 ## Seek further medical advice

Arrange to see your doctor if:

- The infection does not clear up in 2–3 days using the treatment above or from your doctor

 ### DRUG REMEDIES

Antifungal drugs (see p.178) You can use clotrimazole pessaries or cream, which should be introduced into the vagina while you are lying down. Use them at bedtime so they work overnight. Alternatively, take a capsule of fluconazole or use a combination tablet and cream product.

 ### NATURAL REMEDIES

Sodium bicarbonate (see p.188) can help to soothe soreness and irritation. Add 2 tablespoonfuls to a lukewarm, shallow bath.

Live yoghurt contains bacteria that help fight the infection. To insert yoghurt into your vagina, put some in the top of a tampon applicator, then insert the tampon into the vagina. Remove it an hour later.

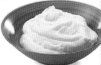

Using yoghurt
Apply it to your vulva and inside your vagina.

 ### PREVENTION

Avoiding attacks If you often have thrush, the following steps may help to prevent recurrences.

- Use only water and unperfumed soap on your genitals. Rinse and dry well after bathing.
- Use only sanitary towels during periods. If you have to use tampons, change them at least every 4 hours.

Genital irritation

Itching inside the vagina or around the vulva (the folds of skin outside the vagina) may be uncomfortable and embarrassing during the day and make it difficult for you to sleep at night. The area may be dry, red, and swollen and you may have a stinging sensation when you pass urine and/or discomfort during sex. Symptoms are usually worse in hot weather. Genital irritation is often a reaction to soaps and perfumes in toiletries, but it can also be due to an infection, another skin condition, or to not drying yourself properly after using the toilet.

 See also Vaginal discharge, opposite page; **Painful intercourse**, p.134.

 ## See your doctor first

Make an appointment to see your doctor if:

- You have a discharge, or pain passing urine
- You have itching elsewhere and/or have a skin condition such as eczema or psoriasis
- You are losing weight without trying and/or are drinking or urinating more than usual
- You have black specks in your pubic hair

What you can do yourself

Try the following home treatments to help relieve itching and reduce inflammation.

- Use a cold compress. Wrap a pack of frozen peas or crushed ice in a wet towel, or soak a face cloth in cold water, then wring it out. Apply it gently to your vulva, as often as needed. You could also sit in a shallow, cool or lukewarm bath for 10–15 minutes.

 • Try a moisturizing cream or ointment to soothe the inflamed skin (*see* DRUG REMEDIES, right).

 • Take a sedative antihistamine to reduce irritation and help you sleep (*see* DRUG REMEDIES, right).

• Use a vaginal lubricant if your vagina feels dry or sore during sex (*see* DRUG REMEDIES, right).

• Resist the urge to scratch your vulva. In bed, wear a nightgown without underwear to let the air circulate around your genital area.

Seek further medical advice

Arrange to see your doctor if:

- Irritation persists for more than 3–4 days

 ### DRUG REMEDIES

Moisturizers (*see* p.186), such as aqueous cream and emulsifying ointment, soothe irritated skin. Apply a moisturizer to your vulva about 3 times a day, and use it as a substitute for soap when washing.

Antihistamines (*see* p.178) relieve itching. A sedative antihistamine, taken at bedtime, will also make it easier for you to sleep.

Vaginal lubricants (*see* LUBRICATING JELLY, p.185) will help to make sexual intercourse more comfortable. Either use a gel just before intercourse or try a longer-acting vaginal moisturizer.

 ### PREVENTION

Avoiding irritation You can help prevent genital irritation by avoiding possible triggers and taking extra care with personal hygiene.

- Don't use perfumed soaps, bubble baths, vaginal deodorants, or douches. Wash your genital area once or twice a day with plain warm water or an unperfumed soap. Pat yourself dry with a soft towel, or use a hairdryer on a cool setting for a few seconds.
- Put your laundry through an extra rinse and don't use fabric softeners.
- Wipe yourself from front to back after a bowel movement and dry yourself thoroughly after passing urine. Use soft, unbleached, uncoloured toilet paper.
- Ask your partner to use hypoallergenic condoms rather than those coated with a spermicide. Don't use deodorized sanitary pads or panty liners.
- Wear comfortable cotton underwear, and change it daily. Choose tights with a cotton gusset, or stockings. Don't wear tight-fitting jeans.
- Change out of your swimsuit promptly after a swim.

Painful intercourse

Many women experience painful sexual intercourse from time to time. Sometimes, the problem is a physical one: for example, sex is often uncomfortable after childbirth, particularly if you had stitches or a tear, or after the menopause when the vagina is less well lubricated. Vaginal infections and irritations, or simply being constipated, can also play a part. Vaginal dryness due to lack of arousal is often a factor in painful intercourse; in extreme cases, a woman may experience spasms in her vaginal muscles that make penetration difficult or even impossible. Physical symptoms such as these are often due to underlying psychological factors such as anxiety, guilt, or previous experience of painful intercourse.

 ## See your doctor first

Make an appointment to see your doctor if:

* You have deep pelvic pain during intercourse
* Vaginal spasms and/or emotional problems may be contributing to painful intercourse

What you can do yourself

If you find intercourse painful, try to identify the cause and take the following steps as appropriate.

 * Try using a lubricating jelly (*see* DRUG REMEDIES, right) if you suffer from vaginal dryness.

* If a certain sexual position causes pain, try another one. Some women like to be on top, so they can control penetration.

* If you think that vaginal dryness might be due to lack of arousal, talk things through with your partner. Make sure you spend enough time on foreplay. Caressing each other without progressing to full intercourse from time to time will take the pressure off and help you both relax.

* Painful intercourse can make you anxious and more likely to tighten up the next time you try to have sex. You may be able to break this vicious circle by spending more time on foreplay as above, soaking in a warm bath, having a glass of wine, and practising muscle relaxation exercises (*see* PRACTICAL TECHNIQUE, p.21) before you have sex.

* Don't use douches or perfumed toiletries in case they cause vaginal discomfort and irritation.

* If you use tampons, check you have not forgotten to remove one at the end of your last period.

 ### DRUG REMEDIES

Lubricating jelly (*see* p.185) Apply a water-soluble jelly to your vagina before you have sexual intercourse. Alternatively, use a longer-lasting vaginal moisturizer that replenishes moisture over several days.

Using lubricants
Long-acting moisturizers are supplied with an applicator, which is inserted into the vagina. Apply jelly directly from the tube or bottle.

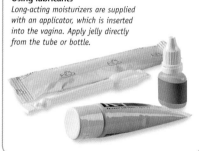

 ## Seek further medical advice

Arrange to see your doctor if:

* The pain continues despite treating the cause and using self-help measures
* You develop other symptoms, such as bleeding from the vagina after intercourse

CHILDREN'S PROBLEMS

Fever (children)

A child with a fever has a temperature raised persistently above 37°C (98.6°F). Children develop a fever more easily than adults. Causes may include a minor illness, such as a cold, ear infection, or chickenpox, or simply being overdressed. A feverish child looks bright-eyed and flushed, and the forehead and neck feel hot. Some children feel shivery and tired and have a headache.

 See also Febrile seizures, p.167.

WARNING

Seek immediate medical help if:

- Your child has a headache and stiff neck, is sensitive to bright light, and/or develops a rash (*see* p.150)
- He or she is drowsy, is breathing fast, or has had a seizure

 ## See your doctor first

Arrange to see your doctor promptly if your child also has earache, a rash, or a sore throat.

What you can do yourself

Use the self-help treatments described below to make a feverish child more comfortable.

- Make sure your child gets plenty of rest, although he or she does not need to stay in bed.

 - Give a painkiller to reduce fever (*see* DRUG REMEDIES, right) and keep offering your child plenty of cool drinks.

 - You can get a good idea of your child's temperature by feeling his or her forehead or the back of the neck. If you need an accurate result, use a thermometer (*see* PRACTICAL TECHNIQUE, right).

- Dress your child in light clothing. Don't swaddle the child in blankets, even if he or she feels shivery. Make sure the room is comfortable and not too hot.

 ## Seek further medical advice

Arrange to see your doctor if:

- Your child does not improve within 24 hours
- His or her temperature continues to rise
- He or she develops new symptoms

DRUG REMEDIES

Painkillers Paracetamol (*see* p.187) and ibuprofen (*see* p.184) bring down a fever and relieve pain. If your child does not respond to one of these, you can try the other but don't give both at the same time. Both medications are available in various forms; ask your pharmacist for advice about a suitable product for your child's age.

PRACTICAL TECHNIQUE

Taking a child's temperature Use an easy-to-read digital thermometer, which is placed in your child's mouth or armpit, or an aural sensor thermometer, the tip of which is inserted into the ear. Take a reading every 2–3 hours. Forehead temperature strips are unreliable, and mercury thermometers are no longer recommended.

Aural thermometer
Gently insert the tip for a few seconds. Remove the thermometer to read the display.

Diarrhoea and vomiting (children)

Diarrhoea and vomiting in a child is often due to gastroenteritis, an infection that can be picked up through contact with infected people or from contaminated food or water. Your child may also have abdominal pains, fever, and a headache. Emotional stress or excitement can cause an upset stomach in some children, as can reactions to food or drink, particularly large amounts of fruit or sugar. Children sometimes develop toddler's diarrhoea – watery stools in which bits of food can be seen – due to not digesting food properly. This usually clears up by the age of 3. A child with an illness that causes a fever or cough may vomit without diarrhoea.

 See also Food intolerance, p.113; Food poisoning, p.114.

 ## See your doctor first

Make an appointment to see your doctor if:

- There is blood in your child's stools or vomit
- Your child has sunken eyes, a dry mouth and tongue, has not passed urine for more than 6 hours, or is abnormally drowsy
- Your child gets repeated bouts of diarrhoea

What you can do yourself

If your child has vomiting and diarrhoea the main risk is dehydration, so you need to replace lost fluids.

 • Make sure your child has plenty to drink. If he or she is still vomiting, give frequent sips of water. You can use an oral rehydration preparation to replace lost fluids and salts (*see* DRUG REMEDIES, right).

• When your child feels ready to eat again, start by offering small amounts of his or her usual diet then gradually increase the amount to normal.

• Give your child paracetamol to ease a fever or stomachache (*see* DRUG REMEDIES, right), but don't give over-the-counter antidiarrhoeal medicines.

 ## Seek further medical advice

Arrange to see your doctor if:

- Your child has abdominal pain for more than 3 hours; vomiting has not stopped after 12 hours; or diarrhoea has not stopped after 24 hours
- Your child is refusing drinks

 ### DRUG REMEDIES

Oral rehydration preparations
(*see* p.186) replace water, salts, and sugars lost from diarrhoea and/or vomiting and prevent dehydration. They are available as sachets of powder in different flavours. Make up a sachet with the recommended amount of fresh drinking water.

Paracetamol for children (*see* p.187) will relieve fever and pain due to gastroenteritis.

Rehydration drink
Offer oral rehydration solution instead of, or in addition to, the child's regular drinks.

PREVENTION

Avoiding infection Be scrupulous about hygiene to prevent infection with gastroenteritis or, if your child already has the infection, to stop it from being passed to other family members.

- Wash your hands thoroughly with soap and water before and after handling or feeding your child; before handling food or eating; and after using the toilet. Make sure other family members do the same.
- Use separate towels and flannels for your child if he or she has an infection.
- Clean the toilet regularly, including the seat and handle, with bleach or disinfectant.
- Make sure your child washes his or her hands after playing outdoors or handling pets.

Threadworms

Threadworms most often affect children. You may notice the tiny worms, like threads of cotton, in your child's stools, but usually the first sign is itching around the anus (and vulva in girls) at night when the worms lay eggs. If your child scratches, the area may become sore and your child may pick up eggs on his or her fingers and reingest them or pass them to others. If many worms are present, your child may have stomachache.

 See also Itchy anus, p.118.

See your doctor first

Make an appointment to see your doctor if you are not sure that your child has a threadworm infestation, or if a child under 3 months has threadworms.

What you can do yourself

Threadworm infestation is usually easy to treat at home with medicine and hygiene measures.

● Give your child a threadworm treatment to kill the worms (*see* DRUG REMEDIES, right). Treat all other family members at the same time, even if they don't have symptoms.

● Get your child to wear underpants at night to help prevent scratching.

● Bathe your child, or wash around his or her anus, every morning to remove any worm eggs that have been laid during the night.

● Ensure your child takes particular care with hygiene (*see* PRACTICAL TIPS, right).

● You don't need to keep your child off school or separated from friends, but do remind him or her to be especially careful about personal hygiene while away from home.

● You don't need to treat pets such as cats and dogs: they don't carry threadworms.

Seek further medical advice

Arrange to see your doctor if:

● Your child continues to have symptoms after about 2–3 weeks despite treatment

DRUG REMEDIES

Threadworm treatments (*see* p.189) include the anthelmintic (worm-killing) drug mebendazole, which is the usual treatment for anyone over 2 years old. A single dose should be effective, although a second dose after 2 weeks is sometimes necessary. For babies and young children aged 3 months–2 years, use piperazine and give a repeat dose after 14 days. These drugs kill the worms but not their eggs, so be careful about hygiene for at least 3 weeks following treatment.

CAUTION: If you are pregnant or breastfeeding, or for babies under 3 months, consult your doctor before using these treatments.

PRACTICAL TIPS

Essential hygiene Be scrupulous about hygiene to break the worm's lifecycle, and to prevent reinfestation and spread to other people.

● Ensure your child washes his or her hands before eating or handling food, and after using the toilet. Keep nails short and discourage finger-sucking and nail-biting.
● Eggs can survive for up to 3 weeks on items such as bedlinen and towels, so change these daily. Don't shake them out because you may spread the eggs. Wash items in hot water and dry them in a tumble-dryer. Give your child a face cloth and towel for his or her own use.

Treating nails
Scrub under the nails to remove any eggs that may be lodged there.

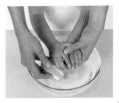

Croup

Croup is a viral infection normally affecting children between 3 months and 3 years old. It usually begins with symptoms such as a runny nose, sneezing, and fever. After a day or two, the child develops a barking cough, like a sea lion, and a hoarse voice. Attacks of croup often occur in the early hours of the morning, and if severe, the child makes a whistling noise (stridor) when breathing in. Most children recover in a couple of days, but the cough may take several days longer to clear up.

> **WARNING**
>
> Seek immediate medical help if:
> - Your child's breathing is noisy or he or she is having difficulty breathing, speaking, or swallowing
> - Your child is drooling, or his or her lips or mouth look blue

See your doctor first

Arrange to see your doctor promptly if you think your child has croup, to confirm the diagnosis and get advice on treatment.

What you can do yourself

While following your doctor's advice, try the following measures to relieve the symptoms.

- Sitting upright will make it easier for your child to breathe. Sit a baby with croup in a baby seat.

- Give paracetamol or ibuprofen to bring down a fever (*see* DRUG REMEDIES, right). Don't give cough medicines.

- Humidify the air in your bathroom and sit there with your child until his or her breathing eases (*see* PRACTICAL TECHNIQUE, right).

- If you are able to, sleep in the same room as your child so you can keep an eye on his or her breathing.

- Encourage your child to rest and take frequent cool drinks during the day.

- Make sure nobody in the home smokes.

Seek further medical advice

Arrange to see your doctor urgently if:

- Your child is still distressed after you have taken steps to treat an attack of croup
- Your child has not recovered from croup after 2 or 3 days of treatment

PRACTICAL TECHNIQUE

Humidifying the air It may help to ease your child's breathing if he or she breathes the moist air in a steamy bathroom. You should sit with your child in the bathroom for about 20 minutes. You may want to take something such as a story or picture book into the bathroom to distract your child.

- Close the bathroom door, run the hot taps into the bath or run the shower, and let the room steam up.
- Sit with your child seated on your knee, supporting his or her back. Stay with your child all the time and make sure he or she keeps clear of the hot water.
- Let your child breathe in the moist air for 15–20 minutes, until his or her breathing gets easier. If this does not relieve symptoms, get immediate medical help.

Breathing steam
Keep your child sitting upright and encourage him or her to take slow, deep breaths.

DRUG REMEDIES

Paracetamol (*see* p.187) and ibuprofen (*see* p.184) are available in various forms and will help reduce fever in croup. Ask your pharmacist to recommend a suitable product for your child's age.

Bedwetting

Although most children become reliably dry at night between the ages of 3 and 7, bedwetting (enuresis) is a common problem for young children. Around 1 in 6 still wet the bed at 5 years; around 1 in 20 are still wetting at age 10. Your child may need treatment if he or she continues after age 7, or starts again after 6 months or more of dry nights. If your child wets the bed regularly, it is most likely to be because he or she has not yet learned bladder control; this will improve in time. Bedwetting is rarely caused by a physical or psychological problem, although a child who has been dry at night may have lapses due to a urine infection or an emotional upset such as bullying; constipation may also be a contributory factor. Bedwetting tends to run in families.

 ## See your doctor first

Make an appointment to see your doctor if:

● You are concerned about bedwetting, especially if your child is over 7 years old or has previously been dry at night
● Your child has a fever and a burning feeling when passing urine, and needs to frequently
● You think your child may be constipated

What you can do yourself

Most children grow out of bedwetting eventually, but in the meantime, try the following steps.

● Never punish your child for bedwetting. Explain to the child that the problem is not his or her fault.

● Don't restrict fluids, but ask your child not to drink anything within 2 or 3 hours of bedtime. Avoid giving chocolate or cola in the early evening.

● Put your child to bed earlier. Make sure he or she uses the toilet before bed. Most bedwetting occurs in the first third of the night, so try waking your child to pass urine before you go to bed.

● Don't put your child in nappies at night, because he or she may not then recognize the need to get up and go to the toilet. Instead, use a waterproof-backed oversheet or plastic mattress cover.

● Try linking your child's progress to rewards. For example, take a jar and give the child a marble to drop in it for every dry night. Offer a reward for a certain number of marbles. Ignore any relapses.

 ● If the above measures have not worked, you could try a pad-and-buzzer alarm system (*see* PRACTICAL TECHNIQUE, right).

 ### PRACTICAL TECHNIQUE

Pad-and-buzzer alarm systems
These systems are sometimes advised for children over 7 years who regularly wet the bed, but they should be used only as a last resort and preferably under medical supervision. They have a moisture-detecting pad which is placed under the bottom sheet, and a buzzer beside the bed. As soon as a child starts to pass urine the buzzer sounds, waking the child so he or she can go to the toilet. Over a few months, the child becomes conditioned to wake before the buzzer sounds and becomes dry at night.

Positioning the pad
The pad is placed under the bottom sheet where the child's hips will lie.

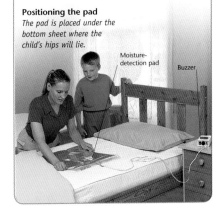

Moisture-detection pad

Buzzer

 ## Seek further medical advice

Arrange to see your doctor if:

● Your child's bedwetting persists despite using the measures described above

Earache (children)

Earache is a common childhood complaint often caused by an infection in the middle ear or the outer ear (swimmer's ear). A build-up of fluid behind the eardrum after a cold or a foreign object pushed into the ear can also cause earache. Sometimes the pain is referred from a sore throat or tooth problem. A young child may not be able to say what is wrong but may pull at one ear; have reduced hearing; be distressed; and be feverish if there is an infection. A discharge from the ear may indicate that the eardrum has burst.

 See also Swimmer's ear, p.65; Popping ears, p.66; Foreign object in the ear, p.68.

 ## See your doctor first

Make an appointment to see your doctor if your child has earache to confirm the diagnosis and be advised on treatment.

What you can do yourself

While following your doctor's advice, there are several measures that you can take to relieve your child's earache. The problem can be very upsetting, especially for young children, so you need to calm your child and distract him or her from the pain.

- Sit your child upright, resting on pillows, as this position may help reduce pressure in the middle ear. Your child will probably sleep better propped up on pillows in bed.

 - Holding a warm towel or well-covered hot-water bottle against the affected ear can help to soothe the pain (*see* PRACTICAL TIP, right).

 - Give your child a painkiller if earache is causing distress (*see* DRUG REMEDIES, right).

- If your child's eardrum bursts, gently wipe away the discharge, keep the ear dry, and have it checked by the doctor.

- Don't poke cotton-wool buds into your child's ear to try to clean it, or insert eardrops or oil unless advised to do so by your doctor.

- Distract your child by reading stories or by playing favourite games.

- Keep your child away from tobacco smoke.

- Offer your child plenty of fluids to drink.

 ### PRACTICAL TIP

Applying warmth Gentle heat can help to relieve earache. Use a well-wrapped hot-water bottle or heat a towel on a radiator or iron it. Check that it is not too hot, then hold it against the affected ear. For a baby, hold a warm, soft cloth over the ear.

Heat treatment
Resting the painful ear on a covered hot-water bottle for about 20 minutes can soothe earache.

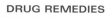

 ### DRUG REMEDIES

Painkillers will help to bring down a fever and reduce the pain of earache. Use one of the various types of paracetamol (*see* p.187) or ibuprofen (*see* p.184) that are formulated specially for children. Your pharmacist will be able to advise which type is most suitable for your child.

Seek further medical advice

Arrange for your child to see your doctor if:

- The earache becomes more severe, or your child is not beginning to feel better after 1–2 days of using treatment from your doctor
- You are concerned that your child's hearing has not returned to normal following treatment

Temper tantrums

Most parents of young children have some experience of temper tantrums. When a child feels frustrated, tired, hungry, or overstimulated he or she may rage, cry, scream, and stamp, kicking and hitting out at anyone or anything close by. Some children vomit, or more rarely, hold their breath to the point of fainting. Tantrums start some time after 1 year, reach a peak between 2 and 3, and usually stop by 4 years. They are part of normal development, but avoiding triggers (such as the child being overtired) will make them less frequent.

 ## See your doctor first

Make an appointment to see your doctor if:

- Your child is having breath-holding attacks
- Your child hurts him- or herself or others during temper tantrums

What you can do yourself

During a tantrum, use the following tips to calm the situation and cope with it constructively.

- At the first signs of a tantrum, try to find and deal with the cause. For example, offer a snack if you suspect your child is hungry, or read a story if he or she seems exhausted but too agitated to sleep. Give the child your undivided attention if possible.

- Even if there is no obvious cause for a tantrum, don't get angry. Shouting and smacking will frighten your child and make the behaviour worse. Show that you still love your child in spite of the tantrum.

- During a full-blown tantrum, it may be hard to get through to your child. As long as the child is in a safe place and not harming him- or herself or others, it may be better to let the tantrum run its course. Stay where your child can see you.

- If a tantrum happens in a public place, ignore the reaction of other people and try to remove or deal with your child calmly and goodhumouredly.

- Don't give in to unreasonable demands or buy your way out of trouble with treats. This will make it more difficult to deal with the next tantrum.

- Breath-holding is usually harmless. During an attack, lay your child flat on the ground. If the child passes out, stay calm; he or she will quickly regain consciousness. If there is any delay or you are concerned, however, seek immediate medical help.

PREVENTION

Avoiding triggers for tantrums

If your child is prone to temper tantrums, it helps to identify situations and frustrations that trigger them. Avoiding them may prevent some tantrums or at least make them milder and less distressing.

- Don't ignore your child. If you are engrossed in other activities, such as speaking on the phone or trying to finish some work, take a break.
- Have reasonable expectations. Notice and reward positive behaviour in your child and ignore minor negative behaviour. Don't fight over trivial matters.
- Save a firm "no" for things that are important, such as safety issues or behaviour that causes potential harm to the child or to others.
- Give your child some control by offering choices instead of instructions. Limit the choices to a simple "either/or" for a young child, such as "Would you like to wear your shoes or your sandals?" or "Would you like to go to the park or play in the garden?"
- Try to keep to regular meals, sleep, and playtimes to prevent your child from becoming hungry or overtired. If there is a change in the daily schedule, prepare your child by explaining as much as can be understood and by ensuring that the child has a favourite item such as a toy or book.
- Young children are often frustrated because they cannot express themselves. Talk to, listen to, and watch your child carefully so you are tuned in to his or her needs, likes, and dislikes.

 ### Seek further medical advice

Arrange to see your doctor if:

- You cannot cope with your child's tantrums
- Tantrums and breath-holding attacks continue after the age of 4

PROBLEMS IN BABIES

Fever (babies)

A baby with a fever has a temperature that is raised persistently above 37°C (98.6°F). He or she may look flushed, and the forehead, back of the neck, and body will feel hot, although the hands and feet may be cold. The baby may be irritable and refuse feeds. Fever is often due to an infection such as a cold, or to being overdressed or too hot. Mild fever after immunizations is also common.

 See also Febrile seizures, p.167.

WARNING

Seek immediate medical help if:
- Your baby's breathing is fast or laboured, or he or she is drowsy
- Your baby has had a convulsion
- Your baby has a red rash that does not fade when pressed (*see* p.150)

 See your doctor first

Arrange to see your doctor promptly if:

- Your baby is under 6 months old
- An older baby is not feeding and/or has vomiting and diarrhoea or a rash, or you are in any way concerned about your baby

What you can do yourself

You should be able to reduce a fever using the following steps, although a mild fever can often be left to run its course if your baby is otherwise well.

- Undress your baby down to a nappy and vest to cool him or her down. Don't overdress your baby or swaddle him or her in blankets – babies can overheat if dressed or covered too warmly.

- Take your baby's temperature (*see* PRACTICAL TECHNIQUE: TAKING A CHILD'S TEMPERATURE, p.135).

- Give paracetamol or ibuprofen to reduce your baby's temperature (*see* DRUG REMEDIES, right).

- Give your baby cooled, boiled water in a bottle in between bottle feeds. If you are breastfeeding, try to increase the length or frequency of feeds.

- Make sure your baby's room is at a comfortable temperature. Use an electric fan if the room is hot.

- Sponging or bathing a baby with tepid water is no longer recommended as it may worsen a fever.

DRUG REMEDIES

Paracetamol (*see* p.187) or ibuprofen (*see* p.184) can be given in liquid form to reduce fever in babies more than 3 months old, and weighing more than 5kg for ibuprofen. For babies 2–3 months old, paracetamol can be given, but only to reduce a fever after immunization. If your baby spits the medicine out, try using a syringe to introduce it slowly.

Medicine syringe
Gently squirt the medicine into the inside of your baby's cheek, not the back of the mouth.

Seek further medical advice

Arrange to see your doctor if:

- Your baby is not getting better within 24 hours, or his or her temperature continues to rise despite the measures described above
- Your baby develops new symptoms

Diarrhoea and vomiting (babies)

Many babies normally have semi-liquid faeces, and regurgitate small amounts of milk after a feed, but diarrhoea and vomiting are more serious. An affected baby passes runny faeces more frequently than normal and may vomit whole feeds. The most common cause of prolonged diarrhoea and vomiting is gastroenteritis (inflammation of the stomach and intestines), which mainly affects bottle-fed babies. Although it usually clears up quickly, there is a risk of your baby becoming dehydrated.

> **WARNING**
>
> Seek immediate medical help if:
> • Your baby is under 3 months old
> • Your baby has blood- or green-stained vomit; bloody or tarry stools; sunken eyes; dry mouth and tongue; dry nappies; or is drowsy

 See also Feeding problems, pp.144–145.

What you can do yourself

There are several steps you can take to relieve mild diarrhoea and vomiting. The main risk is dehydration, so it is important to replace lost fluids.

 • If you are breastfeeding, don't stop. Offer your baby more frequent feeds. If diarrhoea worsens, give your baby an oral rehydration preparation after each feed (*see* DRUG REMEDIES, right).

 • If bottle-feeding, continue full-strength feeds but give smaller amounts more frequently. Offer an oral rehydration preparation (*see* DRUG REMEDIES, right) instead of feeds if your baby refuses formula, or as well as feeds if diarrhoea worsens. Increase fluids gradually; giving too much may encourage vomiting.

• If your baby is taking solids, keep to a normal diet if he or she feels like eating. If your baby has no appetite or continues to vomit, the most important thing is to keep giving fluids. When your baby feels like eating again, offer small amounts of bland foods such as apple purée, mashed banana, and mashed potatoes. Gradually build up the quantities and variety as your baby improves, returning to a normal diet as soon as he or she can tolerate it.

 ## Seek further medical advice

Arrange to see your doctor if:

• Your baby's condition is getting worse
• Your baby is not taking fluids
• He or she has had diarrhoea for 24 hours, or has been vomiting for longer than 3 hours

DRUG REMEDIES

Oral rehydration preparations
(see p.186), available from your pharmacist, are designed to replace water, sugar, and salts lost from diarrhoea and vomiting and to prevent dehydration. They are available as powder in sachets and in different flavours. Make up a sachet with the recommended amount of cooled, boiled water.

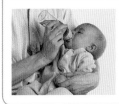

Rehydration
Give your baby rehydration solutions in a bottle to help prevent dehydration.

PREVENTION

Be scrupulous about hygiene
This will help to prevent your baby from getting gastroenteritis or, if he or she has the infection, will stop it from being passed to other family members.

• Wash your hands thoroughly with soap and water before and after handling or feeding your baby; before handling food or eating; and after using the toilet. Make sure everyone in the family does the same.
• Use separate towels and face cloths for your baby if he or she has an infection.
• Wash your baby's hands after he or she has been playing outdoors or handling pets.

Feeding problems

Most feeding problems in babies occur in the early months. Some newborns need practice at latching on to the breast, while bottle-fed babies may have trouble with different sizes of teats and types of formula. Babies who are not getting enough milk are often excessively sleepy and slow to gain weight, while those who are overfed gain weight too quickly. Many breastfed and bottle-fed babies effortlessly posset small amounts of milk after a feed; this is not a cause for concern. Some, however, regurgitate larger amounts of feed and may be wheezy. This condition, called reflux, may last for up to a year and is due to a weak muscle at the entrance to the stomach. It is most common in pre-term babies or those whose muscle tone is poor. A baby who feeds well but wakes screaming between feeds may have an allergy to milk.

 See also Cracked nipples, p.126; **Colic**, p.148.

 ## See your doctor first

Make an appointment to see your doctor if:

- Your baby can't feed or won't feed
- Your baby has been feeding well, but has developed problems
- Your baby regurgitates large volumes of milk and/or there is blood in the vomit
- Your baby fails to gain or loses weight

What you can do yourself

Most feeding problems resolve themselves over time, but using the following tips will help. You can be sure that your newborn baby is feeding well if he or she produces 6 or more wet nappies a day, sleeps well, and gains weight at the predicted rate.

- Make sure your newborn baby feeds properly at least 6 times in 24 hours. Don't assume a sleepy baby is simply "content"; wake your baby for feeds if he or she is sleeping for more than 4 hours.

- Babies who gain weight too fast are usually bottle-fed. Ask your health visitor's for advice about how to regulate feeding.

- If your baby possets milk after a feed, change the nappy beforehand so you don't have to disturb your baby too much after he or she has fed. Pause and wind your baby at intervals during the feed, and hold him or her upright on your lap afterwards to allow wind to come up naturally. If you are bottle-feeding, try using a bottle and teat specifically designed to reduce wind.

 ### PRACTICAL TECHNIQUE

Successful breastfeeding It may take a little practice for both you and your baby to get breastfeeding right. These simple steps will help.

- Hold your baby with the head cradled in the crook of your arm, the bottom well supported and the arm tucked around your body. Whenever possible, have skin to skin contact with your baby during feeds.
- Stroke your baby's cheek with a finger or your nipple so the mouth opens wide and your baby turns towards the nipple. Expressing a little milk on to the nipple will help to encourage your baby.
- Aiming your nipple at the roof of the baby's mouth, make sure the nipple and as much of the areola around it as possible is taken into the mouth. When the baby closes his or her mouth it will form a tight seal.
- If your baby sucks only on the end of the nipple, he or she will not be getting milk and your nipple may become sore. Ease the baby off the breast by gently inserting a finger into the corner of the mouth and reposition him or her to try again.

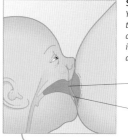

Sucking position
Your baby should take the entire nipple and most of the surrounding areola into his or her mouth during breastfeeding.

The nipple is drawn to the back of the mouth

The jaws press on the areola to pump milk

What you can do yourself *continued...*

- A baby who has been diagnosed with reflux needs a special feeding regime until he or she grows out of the condition (*see* PRACTICAL TIPS, right).

Breastfeeding

- If you have not breastfed before, there are several tips that will help get you off to a good start (*see* PRACTICAL TECHNIQUE, left). Make sure you have help from someone who has had experience in breastfeeding.

- Your baby may find it hard to latch on if your breasts are engorged or very full. Expressing a little milk before he or she begins to feed will soften the breast. This will also help if your baby chokes because your milk flows too fast.

- Until your baby has learned to breastfeed properly, don't use dummies or bottles.

- Occasionally expressing milk by hand or using a breast pump between feeds will help to empty the breast and stimulate a good supply of milk. This also helps to draw out a flat or inverted nipple, as does wearing a nipple shield.

- Make sure you eat an extra 500 calories a day and rest whenever you can to maintain a good milk supply for your baby.

- If your baby is unsettled and wakes screaming between feeds, try excluding dairy products from your diet for a week to see if the problem is due to an allergic reaction to them. If symptoms improve, continue these measures.

Bottle-feeding

- If your baby is feeding too slowly, try a teat with a larger hole. Conversely, a baby who gulps and feeds fast may need a teat with a smaller hole.

- Try changing to a different milk formula if your baby is consistently unsettled or unhappy after feeding. If he or she wakes screaming between feeds, try a hypoallergenic formula for a week to see if the problem is due to milk allergy. If symptoms improve, continue these measures.

- If your baby has diarrhoea and vomiting (*see* p.143), be careful about washing your hands before a feed and be meticulous about sterilizing bottles and equipment.

PRACTICAL TIPS

Coping with reflux A baby with reflux will dislike being laid flat on his or her back and needs to be handled carefully after a feed. The following measures will help to reduce regurgitation.

- Change your baby's nappy before the feed and handle your baby gently and hold him or her upright after the feed.
- Give smaller feeds more frequently to avoid overloading your baby's stomach.
- If you are bottle-feeding, use a thickened formula, designed for babies with reflux problems. (Ask your health visitor or doctor for advice.) Don't add extra powdered formula to a feed. A breastfed baby over 4 months old can be given 2 teaspoonfuls (10 ml) of baby rice dissolved in 2 tablespoons (30 ml) of expressed milk or formula before feeds.
- Your baby may be more comfortable in a baby seat immediately after a feed. Raising the head of the cot slightly on books or bricks may help to make your baby more comfortable during sleep.

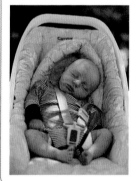

Preventing reflux
Keep your baby semi-upright in a baby chair or seat for the first 30 minutes or so after each feed.

 Seek further medical advice

Arrange to see your doctor if:

- Your baby appears lethargic or listless or you have concerns about his or her weight
- Your baby has symptoms of milk intolerance or allergy, such as diarrhoea, vomiting, abdominal pain, and colic
- Reflux persists after the age of 18 months

Sleep problems (babies)

In the first 3 months of a baby's life, night-waking is to be expected because all babies need to be fed at night. Some continue to need night feeds for up to 6 months. Sleep problems in these early months tend to centre on getting a baby to settle again after a feed, particularly at night, or the baby waking again after a short time. Older babies who are difficult to put to bed and/or who wake at intervals during the night need a fixed bedtime routine and, sometimes, a period of training in how to fall asleep by themselves and resettle themselves when they wake. Illness, changes in routine, and feeding problems can all affect a baby's sleep temporarily.

 See also Feeding problems, pp.144–145; Colic, p.148; Excessive crying, p.149.

See your doctor first

Arrange to see your doctor if:

- Your baby seems unwell or you are concerned about him or her in any way
- Your baby wakes up suddenly screaming and cannot be consoled

What you can do yourself

Try some or all of the following measures if your baby does not sleep well. Sticking to a routine with your baby and being consistent in your approach will bring results, although it may take time.

Babies up to 4 months
- Keep a sleep diary for a week, noting when and how your baby falls asleep and wakes. This will show whether there is a pattern to sleep disturbance and help you decide which strategies might work.

- Put your baby to sleep on his or her back, on a firm mattress with no pillow, towards the foot of the cot, so the bedding cannot cover his or her face.

- Check your baby is not too hot or too cold. Keep the room at about 18°C (65°F) and don't put the cot close to a heater. Don't wrap your baby tightly. Cover him or her with one or two light blankets. Don't use a quilt.

- When your baby wakes for a night feed, keep the lighting low and change the nappy first or do not change it all unless your baby is very wet or has nappy rash. If your baby falls asleep at the breast or bottle, gently replace him or her in the cot. Don't make elaborate attempts to wind the baby or you may wake him or her up again.

PRACTICAL TIPS

Establishing sleep associations
Using the same sequence of events every night will help your baby associate them with falling asleep.

- Bathe your baby at the same time each evening and make this a calm, quiet time, if possible, without too much stimulation and excitement.
- For a baby under 6 months, place the baby on his or her back in an airy cot. Stay beside the cot with your hand resting lightly on his or her chest and sing. Stick to the same song every night as this will now become your baby's sleep association.
- For older babies, sit by the cot spending time with your baby with a book or favourite toy and then settle your baby. Over time, a favourite soft toy, muslin cloth, or blanket may become a transitional object that helps a baby to sleep. Some babies find their own thumb and suck it for comfort.

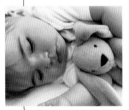
Transitional object
When a baby begins to associate security and comfort with a favoured blanket or soft toy, it becomes a transitional object that helps him or her to sleep.

What you can do yourself *continued...*

- You may want to have your baby in bed with you in the early months, especially if you breastfeed, but be aware of the following precautions. You need a wide, firm bed and to lay the baby on the mattress (not on a pillow) with only a light blanket as a cover. Don't sleep with your baby if you or your partner are smokers, have been drinking alcohol, or have taken sleeping pills or other drugs.

- Try to establish good sleep associations early on (*see* PRACTICAL TIPS, opposite page). Carrying and rocking, or a ride in the pram or car, will help to settle a young baby between feeds during the day, but don't use these methods continually or your baby may not be able to sleep without them.

- Encourage longer sleeps at night by establishing the difference between day and night. Keep the curtains open during daytime naps, and play and chat to your baby while you feed and change him or her. Keep the room dark at night and all stimulation to a minimum during and after a feed.

Babies over 4 months
- Try to establish regular daytime naps because learning to settle and sleep in the day can improve your baby's sleep at night. All babies under a year need two naps of an hour or more each day. Make sure the last nap is early in the afternoon so it does not interfere with sleep at night.

- If your baby is over 4 months and gaining weight and feeding well, you can teach him or her to sleep better at night. A period of night-time training using controlled crying or gradual withdrawal (*see* PRACTICAL TIPS, right) will stop your baby's sleep problems becoming entrenched. Accept that if you have always comforted your baby promptly when he or she wakes, you are sure to feel anxious about this process at first.

- If your baby over 6 months has partial wakenings in which he or she cries briefly and thrashes about, check your baby is safe and well and resettle him or her. Keeping to a routine and preventing overtiredness may help to prevent the problem.

Seek further medical advice

Arrange to see your doctor if:

- Sleep problems are persisting or any unexplained symptoms develop

PRACTICAL TIPS

Controlled crying You can use this technique to teach an older baby (who no longer needs to be fed during the night) to fall asleep at bedtime and to settle again if he or she wakes during the night. You may find the process tough for the first few nights, but for success try to see it through.

- When your baby cries don't rush in; wait for 5 minutes, then enter the room and say "good night" or "back to sleep now" (choose your own phrase). Then leave, even if your baby is still crying.
- Wait for 10 minutes before you return to your baby and repeat the phrase again in a calm, cheerful tone. Repeat the sequence again after a 15-minute interval, then again after a maximum interval of 20 minutes.
- Now restart the procedure entering the room at 5-, 10-, 15-, and 20-minute intervals. Don't give up if your baby continues to cry. Parents need to support each other through this process as most babies protest vigorously at first.
- Use the same technique consistently each night; it should begin to have an effect within 3–6 days.

Gradual withdrawal If you find controlled crying too difficult, try a separation technique called "gradual withdrawal".

- Place your baby awake in the cot, using your settling routine (*see* PRACTICAL TIPS, opposite page) and sit near the cot until your baby falls asleep.
- Every 2–3 days, move the chair a little further from the cot until you are sitting by the door.
- Once you have reached this stage, try settling your baby and leaving him or her to fall asleep alone.

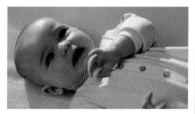

Learning to fall asleep
Your baby may cry vigorously at being left for the first few nights, but if you maintain a consistent approach, he or she will learn to fall asleep alone and to resettle if he or she wakes during the night.

Colic

Colic is used to describe bouts of crying and upset behaviour in an otherwise healthy baby. These bouts tend to recur at the same time each day, usually in the early evening, and can last for 3 hours or more. A colicky baby screams and draws up his or her knees, clenches the fists, and appears to have a stomachache. Comforting has little effect. As many as 1 in 5 babies develops colic, usually starting 2–3 weeks after birth, and no one is sure why it occurs. The problem disappears when the baby is about 4 months old and causes no lasting harm, but it is distressing for parents. In a few babies, colic may be due to a cows' milk allergy.

 See also Feeding problems, pp.144–145; Sleep problems, pp.146–147; **Excessive crying**, opposite page.

 ## See your doctor first

Make an appointment to see your doctor if:

- Your baby's behaviour or crying suddenly changes from its normal pattern
- Your baby has a fever, diarrhoea, or vomiting
- There is blood in your baby's faeces
- Your baby is not gaining enough weight

What you can do yourself

Colic varies from one baby to the next, so try a variety of measures to see which helps.

- If you are bottle-feeding, try changing to a hypoallergenic formula for a week to see if the problem is due to a milk allergy. If you are breastfeeding, exclude dairy products from your diet. If colic improves, continue these measures.

- Too much caffeine in breast milk can make a breastfed baby irritable, so reduce your intake of coffee and other caffeinated drinks.

- "Pause and burp" your baby at least twice during each feed, and don't let your baby guzzle. If you are bottle-feeding, check that the hole in the teat is not too large so the baby gulps, or too small so the baby struggles to feed. You may find an "anti-colic" bottle and teat effective.

 - Experiment with different ways of soothing your baby (*see* PRACTICAL TIPS, right).

- Your baby may pick up on your mood if you are tired and tense. Deep breathing exercises (*see* PRACTICAL TECHNIQUE, p.20) may help you to stay calm through a bout of colic.

 ### PRACTICAL TIPS

Calming a colicky baby A colicky baby can be unpredictable so you might need to switch tactics from time to time.

- If your baby is jumpy and oversensitive to stimulation, try a tranquil, orderly bedtime routine, taking time to bathe and feed your baby. Put him or her in a cot in a quiet place, with the lights dimmed.
- Background noise calms some babies, so try putting your baby to sleep with a vacuum cleaner or washing machine running nearby. If your baby can only be calmed by movement, try an outing in the pram or put him or her in a car seat and go for a drive.
- Enlist help from family and friends during difficult evenings. If you are on your own, put the baby in a sling and sing to him or her while you do other tasks.

Soothing actions
You may find that your baby enjoys being rocked or having you sing to him or her.

 ## Seek further medical advice

Arrange to see your doctor or health visitor if:

- You find it difficult to cope with the crying
- You think the problem is not due to colic

Excessive crying

Crying is the way a baby communicates its needs, and most young babies cry intermittently for up to 3 hours a day. The usual causes are hunger, discomfort from a wet or dirty nappy, wind, loneliness, being too hot or too cold, or being overtired. As parents learn to recognize different types of cry and respond quickly, the baby tends to cry less. However, if you have a baby who cries excessively, he or she will sleep much less than the 16–18 hours that is normal for a newborn baby. Your baby may be difficult to feed, soothe, and settle, and leave you feeling inadequate and exhausted. Most babies grow out of excessive crying by the age of 6 months.

 See also Feeding problems, pp.144–145; Sleep problems, pp.146–147; Colic, opposite page.

See your doctor first

Arrange to see your doctor if:

- Your baby's crying sounds unusual and is accompanied by symptoms such as fever

What you can do yourself

Try the following suggestions to help you cope with a crying baby. Every baby is different, so see what works best for yours.

- If it is more than 2 hours since the last feed, offer another feed. Most newborn babies need to be fed every 2–4 hours, day and night. Wind your baby by holding him gently upright on your lap or over your shoulder.

- Change your baby's nappy if it is wet or dirty. You may find your baby becomes calmer if you let him or her kick freely without a nappy for a short time on the changing mat in a warm room.

- Check the back of your baby's neck to make sure he or she is not too hot or too cold. It should be warm and not sweaty, although your baby's hands and feet may be cooler than his or her body. Adjust clothing and covers as necessary.

 - If your baby seems tired but fights sleep, try a settling routine (*see* PRACTICAL TECHNIQUE, right).

- Put a bored or lonely baby in a baby chair so he or she can watch you, or in a sling facing forwards.

- When you feel you can't cope, take the baby for a walk or put him or her in a cot, and have a break. Ask a relative or friend to take over for a few hours, and use the time to rest, or do something you enjoy.

PRACTICAL TECHNIQUE

Settling a baby If your baby is happy in your arms and only cries when placed in the cot, you may need to develop a settling technique.

- Try holding your baby in your arms and singing for a few minutes until he or she relaxes. Then gently place your baby in the cot, keeping your hand on your baby's chest and continue singing.
- Stay by your baby for 10 minutes or so until he or she can lie happily in the cot, then move away. If crying resumes, lift the baby, comfort and cuddle him or her, and try again.

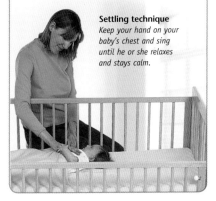

Settling technique
Keep your hand on your baby's chest and sing until he or she relaxes and stays calm.

 ## Seek further medical advice

Arrange to see your doctor if:

- Your baby has developed new symptoms or you are finding it difficult to cope

Spots, rashes, and skin problems

Young babies have sensitive skin that is susceptible to spots and rashes. Most rashes, such as the tiny white spots (milia) seen on the nose and cheeks of newborn babies, are harmless and clear up quickly. However, a rash may be due to a disorder such as eczema, or an infectious illness, such as chickenpox, measles, or meningitis.

 See also Rubella, p.27; Measles, p.29; Chickenpox, p.32; Eczema, p.38; Heat rash, pp.46–47; Nappy rash, p.152.

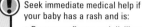
WARNING

Seek immediate medical help if your baby has a rash and is:
- Drowsy or floppy and dislikes being touched or held
- Has a fever, a high-pitched cry, and/or is vomiting or refusing feeds

See your doctor first

Make an appointment to see your doctor if:
- You are unsure what has caused the rash
- Spots are blistered, crusty, or weepy
- A rash is accompanied by other symptoms

What you can do yourself

The measures below will help you identify and deal with your baby's skin problems.

 • A red or purple blotchy rash should be checked carefully (*see* PRACTICAL TECHNIQUE, right).

• Don't use soaps or wipes on your baby until he or she is at least 6 weeks old, as these can dry the skin; use plain water instead. Add a few drops of baby oil to your baby's bath.

• Wash and dry your baby's face carefully after each feed to avoid rashes on the chin or cheeks caused by food traces or regurgitated milk.

• Dress your baby with cotton next to the skin; fabrics such as wool can irritate delicate skin.

• Put a muslin cloth over the undersheet in the pram and cot and change it regularly if your baby dribbles. When holding your baby, use a cloth to prevent his or her skin rubbing against your clothes, and change position occasionally while giving feeds.

 • If a newborn has dry skin on the hands and feet, rub in moisturizing cream (*see* DRUG REMEDIES, right).

 • If your baby develops a heat rash, cool him or her down (*see* PRACTICAL TECHNIQUE: TREATING A BABY WITH HEAT RASH, p.46).

PRACTICAL TECHNIQUE

Checking a rash A dark red or purple blotchy rash may be a sign of meningitis. Using the glass tumbler test will help you to establish whether this is a possibility.

• Press a clear glass firmly against the rash. If the rash does not fade and is still visible through the glass, get medical help immediately.
• If the rash fades, repeat the test again later. In a few cases, a meningitis rash fades at first but later becomes typical and does not fade when pressed.

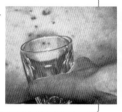

Possible meningitis
This rash is still visible when the glass is pressed against the skin, so it may be a sign of meningitis.

DRUG REMEDIES

Moisturizers (*see* p.186), such as aqueous cream or an unperfumed baby cream, will help moisturize and protect your baby's skin. Apply a cream thinly to the skin after washing your baby.

Seek further medical advice

Arrange to see your doctor if:

- A skin problem does not clear up promptly
- A rash becomes blistered, crusty, or weepy, or your baby develops a fever

Cradle cap

Thick, crusty yellowish scales, known as cradle cap, sometimes develop on a baby's scalp during the first few months of life. The skin may be reddened, and the scales occasionally spread to the baby's forehead and behind the ears. If your baby has hair, you may notice flakes that look similar to dandruff. There is no particular cause for cradle cap, and it is unlikely to bother your baby. However, if he or she has many thick scales, it can look unsightly. Usually, the condition has disappeared completely by the time a baby is 1 year old.

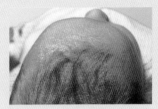
Cradle cap on a baby's scalp

What you can do yourself

Although cradle cap tends to clear up by itself eventually, using these home treatments will help prevent the build-up of scales and improve the appearance of your baby's scalp.

● Wash your baby's scalp every day with a mild baby shampoo, rinse off thoroughly with warm water, then gently dry the scalp with a soft towel.

● After washing your baby's hair, brush the hair and scalp with a soft baby brush to remove the scales. You may find this is enough to clear up a mild case of cradle cap and it will prevent the condition from recurring.

 ● Massaging your baby's scalp with oil will help to remove thick or crusty scales (*see* PRACTICAL TECHNIQUE, right).

 ● For more persistent cradle cap, try a special shampoo for babies that contains coal tar and salicylic acid (*see* DRUG REMEDIES, right).

● Don't try to pick off the scales as this may make your baby's head sore.

✚ Seek further medical advice

Arrange to see your doctor if:

● The cradle cap is not getting better after a few weeks of home treatment
● The scales begin to spread to other areas, such as the baby's neck, armpits, or groin
● The rash or the underlying scalp becomes very red or weepy

PRACTICAL TECHNIQUE

Oil treatment Massaging olive oil or baby oil gently into your baby's scalp with your fingers will help to loosen cradle cap scales. You can leave the oil on for a few hours or overnight, then shampoo it off afterwards. Once your baby's hair has dried, gently brush the hair and scalp with a soft baby brush, and the scales should flake off. Brushing every day may stop the scales forming again.

Scalp massage
Gently rub the oil into your baby's scalp. This will soften loose scales of skin so they can be brushed away more easily.

DRUG REMEDIES

Coal tar and salicylic acid shampoo (*see* ANTI-DANDRUFF SHAMPOOS, p.177) may help to clear cradle cap if your baby has many thick scales of skin on the scalp. Massage a small amount into your baby's scalp, leave it for a few minutes, then wash it out. Shampoo your baby's head again, taking care to rinse the scalp well afterwards.

Nappy rash

Nearly all babies are affected by nappy rash at some time, usually due to urine and faeces irritating the skin where it is in direct contact with the soiled nappy. Leaving a baby in a wet or soiled nappy for too long can cause nappy rash, as can a bout of diarrhoea. Sometimes the rash is a reaction to new foods in the diet. If your baby has nappy rash, the nappy area will look red and sore, and your baby may be irritable. If the rash becomes infected, it may affect the whole nappy area, including the skin creases around the groin. It will then have a red, glistening appearance with pus-filled spots and will be extremely sore.

 ## See your doctor first

Make an appointment to see your doctor if:

- The nappy rash looks infected or the skin is broken, cracked, or bleeding
- Your baby has a fever

What you can do yourself

There are several measures you can take to treat nappy rash and prevent infection. Most cases of nappy rash clear up in 3–4 days.

- Change your baby's nappy often to prevent skin irritation (see PRACTICAL TECHNIQUE, right). Newborn babies will need a nappy change at every feed (at least six a day). While your baby has a rash, change the nappy even more frequently.

- Don't use perfumed skin products or baby wipes, which may contain ingredients that sting sore skin, or soaps, which remove the natural oils from the skin, leaving it more prone to dryness and cracking.

- Wash fabric nappies with a non-biological washing powder and rinse well.

- If your baby has started mixed feeding, introduce one new food at a time to see if anything causes a bout of nappy rash.

 ## Seek further medical advice

Arrange to see your doctor if:

- The rash is not clearing up after a week
- The whole nappy area, including the skin creases, becomes affected, or the skin becomes red and hot and pus-filled spots form

 ### PRACTICAL TECHNIQUE

Nappy changing Adopt this nappy changing routine while your baby has nappy rash to help sore skin heal and prevent recurrences.

- When changing the nappy, first wipe away any faeces using a dry tissue or cotton wool, and then pour or spray warm water over the area and wipe again. Dab dry with a soft towel.
- Let your baby kick without a nappy on the changing mat for about 10 minutes to expose his or her skin to the air. This helps prevent fungal infections.
- Don't use talcum powder when changing nappies.
- Protect your baby's skin by applying a barrier cream, such as zinc and castor oil cream (see DRUG REMEDIES, below) before putting on a fresh nappy.
- Use a high-absorbency nappy that draws away wetness from your baby's skin.

Barrier cream
Apply a thin layer of cream, taking care to protect the skin folds around the top of the legs.

 ### DRUG REMEDIES

Zinc and castor oil cream is often used as a barrier cream to treat and prevent nappy rash. Apply the cream to the nappy area after each wash and nappy change.

FIRST AID

In the following section you will find basic first-aid
techniques for minor problems, such as blisters and insect
stings, and essential instruction to help you deal with
potentially life-threatening injuries and situations, such
as choking and shock. Don't wait for an emergency
before you refer to these pages
because you will be better
equipped if you familiarize
yourself with the basics now.
Although the advice given
here may be invaluable in an
emergency, it is not intended
to be a replacement for the
practical training that is
given on a first-aid course.

First aid essentials

To give first aid effectively, it is important to be well prepared. The step-by-step plan given below can be applied to any emergency to help you deal with a casualty. Cross references take you to the specific first aid techniques you may need on other pages. Access to first aid materials can make all the difference in an emergency, so an essential kit is described here.

> **WARNING**
>
> If you cannot approach a casualty without putting yourself in danger, leave him or her and call the emergency services immediately.

Emergency action plan

The following step-by-step plan will help you deal calmly, safely, and efficiently with a casualty in any situation.

1 Make sure you are safe Before you act, it is important that you and the casualty are not in any danger. Deal with hazards if you can do so safely; if not, call the emergency services.

2 Assess the casualty Check the casualty for life-threatening injuries. If he or she has minor injuries and is alert and talking to you, make sure there are no less obvious injuries. If the casualty does not respond to you, he or she may be unconscious, which is potentially life-threatening. Ask someone to call an ambulance.

3 Check the airway is clear If the airway is blocked and the casualty is conscious, treat choking (*see* p.172); if the casualty is unconscious, open the airway (*see* p.168).

4 Check breathing If the casualty is conscious, treat any breathing difficulties, such as asthma (*see* Wheezing, p.103). If the casualty is unconscious and is not breathing, begin cardiopulmonary resuscitation immediately (*see* CPR, pp170–171); continue until help arrives – do not go to the next step unless the casualty begins breathing normally.

5 Check for bleeding When the casualty is breathing normally, check for any serioius bleeding and, if necessary, treat it by applying direct pressure (*see* p.157).

6 Deal with other injuries When you are certain that the casualty's breathing and circulation are stable, check for and treat any other injuries.

FIRST AID KIT

You can buy a first aid kit or make up your own and put it in an airtight box or tin. Store the kit in a cool, dry place, out of reach of children, but make sure it is easy to access. Store a face cloth and a blanket with the kit and keep an extra first aid kit in the car.

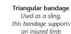

Adhesive dressings
These are used to cover small cuts, grazes, and blisters

Triangular bandage
Used as a sling, this bandage supports an injured limb

Crêpe roller bandages
These apply pressure to a wound or support a sprain or strain

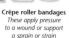

Gauze roller bandages
These bandages are used for holding a dressing in place

Gauze dressing
This is placed directly on a wound and bandaged in place

Wound dressing
This is a sterile dressing attached to a bandage

Tubular bandage and applicator
These are used to dress fingers and toes

Cleansing wipes
Alcohol-free wipes are used to clean wounds when there is no water

Adhesive tapes
Microporous tape or adhesive tape holds dressings in place

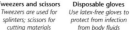

Tweezers and scissors
Tweezers are used for splinters; scissors for cutting materials

Disposable gloves
Use latex-free gloves to protect from infection from body fluids

Cold pack
This helps to reduce swelling in sprains and strains

Blisters

Usually occurring on the feet and hands, blisters are caused by friction or pressure. First the skin becomes red and sore, then fluid collects under the surface in a pale, puffy skin sac. You may get blisters on your heel, sole, or toes from wearing boots or shoes that are badly fitting, or that have not been "broken in". Blisters on the hands are often the result of heavy manual work. Most blisters heal quickly: as new skin grows beneath them, the fluid is reabsorbed and the surface dries and peels away.

 ## Seek medical advice

Arrange to see a doctor if:

- You have blisters that were not caused by friction or pressure and/or you have other symptoms
- A blister becomes red, painful, and swollen, and oozes pus or blood
- You have recurrent blisters or blisters that heal very slowly
- You have diabetes

What you can do yourself

Use the following procedure to treat your blister. Protecting it from further rubbing and friction will help it to heal.

- Don't burst a blister or cut the skin over it. The skin protects against infection.

 - Clean and dry the blister, and protect it with an adhesive dressing or blister plaster (*see* PRACTICAL TECHNIQUE, right).

- If the blister bursts, don't pick at any loose skin around it. Clean, dry, and dress it, as above, and change the dressing daily until it has healed. Leave the area exposed at night to help it dry out.

 ### PRACTICAL TECHNIQUE

Treating a blister
Treat your blister gently to avoid breaking the skin, and keep it clean and dry to reduce the risk of infection.

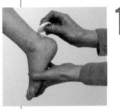

1 *Wash the blister carefully with clean water. Gently pat it dry with a clean cotton pad.*

2 *Cover the blister with an adhesive dressing or blister plaster, making sure that the pad is bigger than the blister. A hydrocolloid plaster absorbs fluid from the blister and cushions it. For large blisters, use a sterile dressing secured with adhesive tape.*

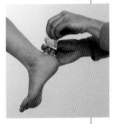

PREVENTION

Avoiding blisters The following tips will help protect feet and hands from friction and pressure.

- Wear well-fitting shoes or boots, and break them in slowly. Put padding such as moleskin pads on areas that are likely to rub and develop blisters.
- If you plan to walk long distances, wear close-fitting synthetic inner socks to prevent friction and a second pair of socks on top.
- Use protective gloves for heavy manual work.

Cuts, grazes, and splinters

Small cuts, grazes, and splinters are common injuries. Cuts usually bleed for a short time. Grazes bleed less, but may be painful and have dust and dirt trapped in them. You can often see or feel splinters in your skin or under nails, or you may not notice them until the area becomes red, hot, and painful due to infection. These injuries, though minor, can carry the risk of tetanus, a serious bacterial infection that can be fatal. People are normally immunized against it in childhood but may need boosters as adults. After treating any injury that breaks the skin, check that tetanus immunization is up to date. Seek medical advice if it is more than 10 years since immunization or if you are not sure when the last injection was given.

PRACTICAL TECHNIQUE

Removing a splinter

Most splinters can be removed easily. Your aims are to remove the entire splinter, if possible, and to minimize the risk of infection. Put on latex-free disposable gloves first, if available, or wash your hands thoroughly.

1 *Clean the area around the splinter with soap and warm water and pat it dry with a gauze pad. Sterilize a pair of tweezers by passing the ends through the flame of a lighter or match. Allow the tweezers to cool down before you use them.*

2 *Squeeze the skin around the splinter to make the end stick out. Grasp the splinter with the tweezers and gently pull it out, at the same angle at which it entered. Try not to break the splinter.*

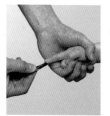

3 *Squeeze the skin around the wound to make it bleed a little; this will flush out any remaining dirt. Clean the area again with warm, soapy water, pat it dry, and cover it with an adhesive dressing.*

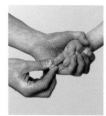

4 *Seek medical advice if a large splinter cannot be removed easily; the site of the splinter becomes hot, red, swollen, and painful; the casualty becomes feverish; and/or the casualty is not up to date with tetanus immunization.*

Treating a small wound or graze

Your main aims when treating a minor cut, graze, or other wound are to control bleeding and minimize the risk of infection. Before you start, put on latex-free disposable gloves, if available, or wash your hands thoroughly.

1 *Control bleeding by pressing a sterile or clean gauze pad firmly on the wound. Raise the injured area above the level of the heart, if possible, to reduce the flow of blood to the wound. Most small cuts will stop bleeding within a few minutes.*

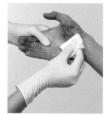

2 *Rinse the wound with cool running water. Clear out as much dirt as you can. Use a gauze pad to clean the surrounding skin. Lift any debris in the wound with the corner of the pad, if necessary.*

3 *Dab the area dry with a clean pad. Cover the wound with an adhesive dressing. Do not use cotton wool or any fluffy material that may stick to the wound.*

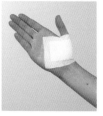

4 *Seek medical advice if the wound is gaping or deeper than was first suspected; you cannot remove gravel or dirt from the wound; the site becomes hot, red, swollen, and painful; and/or the casualty is not up to date with tetanus immunization.*

Severe bleeding

Severe bleeding is likely to be distressing both for the casualty and for the person who is assisting. It is usually the result of a serious injury such as a stab wound, a severe blow, or a deep cut. The main priorities are to stop the bleeding then to monitor the casualty's condition continually. If a large amount of blood is lost, life-threatening shock may develop.

> **WARNING**
> Call an ambulance.
> Profuse or prolonged bleeding can be life-threatening.

PRACTICAL TECHNIQUE

Treating severe bleeding

While you wait for medical help to arrive, your immediate priority is to stem the flow of blood. Once you have done this, you need to dress the wound as quickly as possible to reduce the risk of infection. You then need to check that the bandage is not restricting circulation. As shock (see p.165) is likely to develop, you should lay the casualty down and raise his or her legs to minimize its effects.

1 Put on disposable gloves or wash your hands. Apply pressure on the wound with a clean, non-fluffy pad or the palm of your hand. Raise the injury above heart level to reduce blood loss. If an object is embedded in the wound, don't remove it; press firmly on either side of it to push the edges of the wound together. Call an ambulance.

Keep the injured area raised while you apply pressure

2 Help the casualty to lie down, keeping the injured part raised above the heart. Continue to apply firm pressure on the wound for up to 10 minutes.

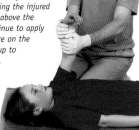

3 Cover the wound with a sterile dressing and secure it with a bandage that is tight enough to maintain pressure but not so tight that it impairs the blood supply.

CAUTION: Do not apply a tourniquet. If there is an object in the wound, build up padding on either side and bandage carefully to avoid pressing on the object.

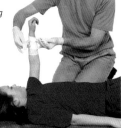

4 Check the circulation beyond the bandage every 10 minutes. Press on a nail or the skin beyond the bandage until it turns pale, then release the pressure. If the colour does not return, or returns slowly, the bandage is too tight. Loosen a tight bandage just a little, making sure the injured part is still supported.

5 If further blood loss occurs, apply a second dressing on top of the first. If blood continues to seep through the top dressing, remove both dressings and apply a fresh one. Bandage firmly, making sure that you are applying pressure accurately over the point of bleeding.

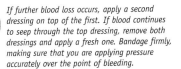

6 Raise and support the casualty's legs above the level of the heart and watch for signs of shock (see p.165). Monitor and record breathing, pulse, and level of consciousness. If the casualty becomes unconscious (see p.168), be prepared to begin CPR (see pp.170–171) if he or she stops breathing.

Insect bites and stings

Wasp, hornet, or bee stings are painful, and the site of a sting may be swollen, red, sore, and itchy for a day or two. Flea and mosquito bites develop into itchy red bumps, while a tick (a tiny bloodsucking creature) leaves a swollen, red, bead-like lump on your skin. Ticks can spread disease so must be removed quickly and carefully. Although most bites and stings are little more than a nuisance, a few people suffer a severe allergic reaction (anaphylactic shock) that needs emergency treatment.

WARNING

Call an ambulance if:
• There are signs of anaphylactic shock (*see* opposite page)
• You suspect the sting is to the inside of the mouth or throat

What you can do yourself

There are effective techniques for removing stings and ticks, and remedies that will reduce the general discomfort of bites and stings.

• Watch for symptoms of anaphylactic shock (*see* opposite page). Call an ambulance if any develop.

• If you suspect a sting to the mouth or throat, call an ambulance. Sucking ice cubes or sipping cold water will help to reduce swelling.

 • To treat a sting, remove the sting, then wash and cool the area (*see* PRACTICAL TECHNIQUE, right).

• If you find a tick, remove it with tweezers. Grasp the head and lever it out, taking care not to leave any of the tick behind. Put the tick in a bottle and see your doctor, taking the tick with you.

• Do not scratch a bite or sting because this will increase the risk of infection.

• Apply an insect bite relief cream or spray (*see* p.184) to soothe sore, swollen, and/or itchy bites.

• Antihistamine tablets (*see* p.178) may help to minimize itching and swelling. You can take medication yourself, but you should not administer it if you are treating someone else.

Seek medical advice

Arrange to see a doctor after 24 hours if:

• Redness and swelling increase
• The bite is oozing or there are red streaks under the skin around the bite

PRACTICAL TECHNIQUE

Treating an insect sting

Follow these steps as soon as possible after the sting has occurred. They will help to reduce immediate pain and swelling and minimize after-effects such as redness, soreness, and itching.

1 *If you are stung on your wrist, hand, or fingers, remove rings, bracelets, and watches in case swelling develops. If the sting is on a limb, keep it raised to reduce swelling. If you cannot see the sting, go to step 3.*

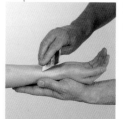

2 *Scrape out a sting that is visible using a firm object, such as a credit card or your fingernail, applying a constant pressure. Don't use tweezers; they may inject more venom into the skin.*

3 *Wash the area with soap and water. Make an ice pack from a bag of frozen peas or crushed ice, wrapped in a towel, or a cloth soaked in cold water and wrung out. Apply it over the site for 10 minutes to reduce pain and swelling.*

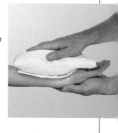

Anaphylactic shock

Certain people develop this life-threatening allergic reaction to insect stings, to some foods such as peanuts or shellfish, or to certain drugs. Anaphylactic shock develops within minutes and causes a sudden drop in blood pressure and narrowing of the airways. Symptoms include wheezing; swelling around the eyes and of the face, lips, and tongue; widespread red, blotchy skin eruptions; gasping for air; and anxiety. There is a risk of shock (see p.165), and the person may become unconscious.

WARNING

Call an ambulance.
A person with anaphylactic shock needs urgent medical attention.

PRACTICAL TECHNIQUE

Treating anaphylactic shock

Your aim is to get the casualty to hospital immediately. A person with anaphylactic shock needs emergency medical help, including an injection of adrenaline (epinephrine). People who are susceptible to this type of allergic reaction often carry a prefilled syringe of adrenaline (epinephrine) for self-treatment, but may need your help to use it. While you wait for specialized help to arrive, you should try to ease the casualty's breathing, watch him or her carefully for any signs of shock, and treat if necessary.

1 *Call an ambulance. Tell the operator that you suspect anaphylactic shock, and give any information you have on what has triggered the reaction. The casualty may be able to give you the details.*

Help the casualty to find and use his or her adrenaline (epinephrine) syringe. The injector can be applied through clothing.

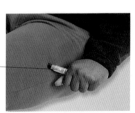

2 *If the casualty is conscious, help him or her into a sitting position to make it easier to breathe. Stay calm and be reassuring. Encourage the casualty to breathe more slowly and deeply. If the casualty becomes pale and/or has a weak pulse, lay the casualty down and raise his or her legs.*

Sitting up will help the casualty to breathe more easily

Support and reassure the casualty until help arrives

3 *If the casualty has a syringe of adrenaline (epinephrine), help him or her to find and use it, or administer it yourself if you know how to do so.*

4 *Monitor breathing, pulse, and level of consciousness until help arrives. Repeat the adrenaline (epinephrine) every 5 minutes if the casualty does not improve or if symptoms return. If the casualty loses consciousness but is breathing, place him or her in the recovery position (see p.169). Be prepared to begin CPR (see pp.170–171) if the casualty stops breathing.*

Sprains and strains

Sprains and strains are common sports injuries. In a sprain, the ligaments around a joint, such as the ankle, are damaged by overstretching. This is often due to a sudden, unexpected wrenching motion that pulls bones too far apart and tears surrounding tissues. In a strain, the muscles or tendons are overstretched and may be partially torn. The symptoms are much the same for both: there will be pain, swelling, and bruising in the injured limb, and it may feel hot and be difficult to move. Sprains and strains are treated in a similar way and normally improve after a few days, but full recovery may take several weeks.

 ## Seek medical advice

Arrange to see a doctor if:

- You have severe pain, or hear a "pop" at the time of the injury
- You can't put weight on a joint or the injured area looks deformed
- You are concerned about the seriousness of an injury

What you can do yourself

You can treat a minor sprain or strain using the following measures. Start the treatment as soon as possible to reduce symptoms and speed recovery.

 - Follow the **R.I.C.E.** procedure (*see* PRACTICAL TECHNIQUE, right).

- Take paracetamol (*see* p.187) to relieve pain or ibuprofen (*see* p.184), which also has an anti-inflammatory effect. You can also gently massage a gel or cream containing ibuprofen into the affected area to reduce pain, but don't use ibuprofen gel if you are already taking ibuprofen by mouth. You can use painkillers to treat yourself, but you should not administer medication if you are treating someone else.

- Keep an elasticated or crepe bandage, on the limb for the first 48 hours, taking it off at night. Once the bandage is removed, you can start moving the limb gently to the limit of pain-free movement. If there is no reduction in pain and swelling after 2–3 days, seek medical advice.

 ### PRACTICAL TECHNIQUE

R.I.C.E. procedure
The mnemonic **R.I.C.E.** stands for **Rest, Ice, Comfortable support,** and **Elevation,** all of which help to speed recovery after a sprain or strain.

1 **Rest** *the injured limb. Avoid any activity that brings on the pain or makes it worse. Sit or lie with the limb in a comfortable position.*

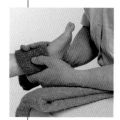

2 **Ice** *reduces pain and swelling. Apply an ice pack (a bag of frozen peas or crushed ice, wrapped in a dry towel or cloth), or a cloth soaked in cold water and wrung out, as soon as possible. Hold for 10 minutes.*

3 **Comfortable support** *involves wrapping padding around the area and securing it with an elasticated or crepe bandage. The bandage should extend from the joint below the injury to the joint above it. Check that the blood flow is not restricted (see Bleeding p.157, step 4).*

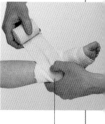
Apply bandage firmly and evenly

4 **Elevation** *reduces blood flow to the area and minimizes bruising. Raise the injured limb on a stool or cushions. Try not to use the limb for the first few hours after injury.*

Fractures and dislocations

A fracture is a break or crack in a bone due to a heavy blow or a sudden twist or wrench. In open fractures, the bone protrudes through the skin; in closed fractures, the skin is not broken. In a dislocation, the bones of a joint are pulled apart. Signs of a broken bone or dislocated joint include swelling, bruising, and deformity at the site of the injury, and pain and difficulty moving the affected part. A serious fracture, for example of the thigh bone, may cause severe internal bleeding and shock (*see* p.165).

> **WARNING**
> Get medical attention immediately if you suspect a broken bone or a dislocated joint. A person who has a broken arm can be taken to hospital by car. Otherwise, call an ambulance.

PRACTICAL TECHNIQUE

Treating a broken arm
Your main aims are to treat any bleeding, support the injury, and arrange transport to hospital. Don't move the casualty until the arm has been immobilized, unless he or she is in danger. Treat dislocations in the same way. Never attempt to manipulate bones back into place.

1 *If the casualty can bend the injured arm, ask him or her to support it. If the bone is protruding from the wound, put on disposable gloves, if available. Cover the wound with a clean dressing. Apply pressure to control bleeding, but don't press on the bone end.*

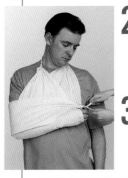

2 *Make a sling using a triangular bandage; tie an extra bandage over the sling to immobilize the arm against the chest. Don't allow the casualty to eat or drink in case an anaesthetic is needed.*

3 *If the casualty cannot bend the arm, put padding around the area and use bandages to immobilize it against the body; don't bandage over the injury site. Call an ambulance.*

Improvised sling
If no sling is available, turn the edge of the casualty's jacket up over the injured arm and attach it to the top of the jacket with a pin.

Treating a broken leg or pelvis
Your main aims are to protect the injured part, call an ambulance, and, for a broken leg, treat any bleeding. Don't move the casualty until the injured part has been immobilized with bandages. Never attempt to manipulate broken bones back into place.

1 *Support joints above and below the injury site. Help the casualty to lie down. Call an ambulance. If a bone is protruding, put on disposable gloves, loosely cover the wound with a dressing, and apply pressure to control bleeding; do not to press on the bone end.*

2 *If the leg is broken, put rolled blankets or coats around the injured leg. Do not let the casualty eat or drink in case an anaesthetic is needed in hospital.*

Put padding around the injured leg

3 *For a broken pelvis, place padding around the body and, if necessary or more comfortable for the casualty, slip a cushion or pillows under the knees.*

4 *If a large bone, such as the thigh bone or pelvis, is broken, treat the casualty for shock (see p.165). Keep the casualty's head low but do not raise the legs. Monitor and record the casualty's breathing, pulse, and level of consciousness. If the casualty becomes unconscious (see p.168), be ready to begin CPR (see pp.170–171) if he or she stops breathing.*

Head injuries

All head injuries are potentially serious. A blow to the head may cause a bruise or scalp injury and sometimes concussion, a brief period of unconsciousness. There is a risk of an underlying skull fracture, as well as compression of the brain from bleeding inside the skull or swelling of injured brain tissues. Symptoms, such as intense headaches, noisy, slow breathing, and drowsiness, may develop hours or even days after the injury. Anyone with a head injury should also be treated for a potential neck (spinal) injury.

> **WARNING**
>
> Call an ambulance immediately if:
> - There is severe bleeding and/or blood or watery fluid is leaking from the ears or nose
> - A casualty loses consciousness

What you can do yourself

You should seek medical advice for all head injuries, even if they are apparently minor.

- For a scalp wound, try to stem any bleeding and dress the injury (see PRACTICAL TECHNIQUE, right).

- If there has been a minor knock to the head but there is no bleeding, apply a cold compress (a towel soaked in cold water and wrung out) to reduce swelling and bruising.

- If the casualty has concussion, he or she may feel sick and dizzy and have a headache. Make sure that the casualty rests, even if he or she seems to have recovered, and seek medical advice.

- If the casualty is conscious but you suspect a more serious head injury, help him or her to lie down in a comfortable resting position. Assume that any casualty with a head injury also has a back or spine injury. Support the head and neck and don't let the casualty move them. Ask simple questions. If the casualty seems confused or has difficulty speaking, call an ambulance.

- If the casualty becomes unconscious (see p.168), call an ambulance. Monitor the casualty's pulse, breathing, and level of response regularly until medical help arrives.

- If the casualty stops breathing, lift the jaw very carefully to open the airway and begin CPR (see pp.170–171).

- After a head injury, watch for symptoms such as headaches, weakness, unequal pupil size, and confusion in the hours and days after the injury. Seek immediate medical help if symptoms develop.

PRACTICAL TECHNIQUE

Treating a scalp wound

Bleeding from a scalp wound is often profuse because the area has many small blood vessels. For this reason, a scalp injury may look more serious than it is. If you are in any doubt about the severity of a wound, seek medical advice.

1 *Wear disposable gloves if available, or wash your hands thoroughly. Cover the injury with a clean pad or sterile dressing, pressing firmly on the wound to control the bleeding.*

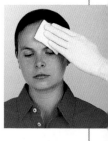

2 *Bandage the dressing in place. If blood seeps through, put a second dressing on. If bleeding continues, remove both dressings and apply a fresh one. Help the casualty into a half-sitting position. Monitor breathing, pulse, and consciousness; watch for shock (see p.165).*

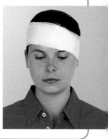

Eye injuries

Eyes are easily bruised or cut by direct blows. They can also be damaged by sharp objects such as fragments of glass, or irritated by grit or dust entering the eye. Chemical splashes may harm the eyes, and many household products, such as detergents, cause irritation if they come into contact with the eyes. An eye injury is usually painful, and the affected eye may water and look swollen and bloodshot. All eye injuries are potentially serious, because there is a risk that vision will be affected.

> **WARNING**
>
> Get emergency medical help if:
> - An eye injury causes loss of vision or blurred vision
> - An object is embedded in the eye
> - A chemical has splashed the eye
> - A child has an eye injury

PRACTICAL TECHNIQUE

Treating eye injuries

You should seek medical advice for all but the most minor eye injuries. Your main aims are to keep the casualty calm, dress the wound, and get medical help.

1 *Examine the eye carefully. If the casualty has a black eye, and you are sure that the injury is not more serious, you may be able to treat it (see p.62). A foreign object in the eye, such as a speck of dirt or debris, can be removed as long as it is floating freely on the white of the eye (see p.61).*

CAUTION: Don't try to remove debris from the coloured part of the eye or remove anything embedded in the eye.

2 *If the eye has been badly cut or bruised, help the casualty to lie down and rest his or her head in your lap to keep it still. Tell him or her to try to keep the eyes still. Cover the injured eye with a sterile dressing or clean pad, and ask the casualty to hold it in place. Arrange for medical help.*

Treating chemicals in the eye

You must act quickly to wash the chemical out of the casualty's eyes. Protect yourself and make sure that the contaminated water drains away freely.

1 *Put on protective gloves, if available. Hold the eye under gently running cold water for at least 10 minutes, positioning the head so that contaminated water does not run into the other eye or down the face. Rinse the eye and eyelid thoroughly. If both eyes are affected, tilt the head to the other side and repeat the procedure.*

Rinse the eye thoroughly

2 *Once the pain has eased, give the casualty a sterile dressing or clean pad to hold lightly over the eye. Bandage the dressing loosely in place if hospital treatment will be delayed. Take or send the casualty to hospital. Identify the chemical if possible so hospital staff can be informed.*

Burns and scalds

Most minor burns occur in the home – for example, after touching a hot oven or spilling hot water. The skin turns red and the burn feels sore. Deeper burns tend to blister and are usually swollen and painful. Severe burns, which damage deeper layers of skin and sometimes the fat and nerves underneath, may look grey and charred. There may be little or no pain. They cause fluid loss and may lead to shock (*see* opposite page).

WARNING

Call an ambulance if:
- A burn is near the mouth or throat, or is extensive or deep
- There are signs of shock, breathing problems, or a casualty becomes unconscious

Seek medical advice

Arrange to see a doctor if:

- A child has a burn
- A burn is on the hands, face, feet, or genitals
- You are unsure about the severity of a burn
- The burn is an electrical or chemical burn

What you can do yourself

For both minor and more serious burns, act quickly to make the casualty safe and cool the burn.

Severe burns
- Move the casualty away from the source of the heat as quickly as you can.

- Cool the burn immediately by flooding it with cold water (*see* PRACTICAL TECHNIQUE, right).

- Watch the casualty carefully for symptoms of shock (*see* opposite page) and treat if necessary. If the casualty becomes unconscious (see p.168), be ready to start CPR (see pp.170–171) if he or she stops breathing.

- Take or send the casualty to hospital.

Minor burns

- Cool the burn immediately by flooding it with cold water (*see* PRACTICAL TECHNIQUE, right).

- While a burn is healing, don't break any blisters that appear. Take paracetamol (*see* p.187) or ibuprofen (*see* p.184) if the burn is still painful.

- If a burn itches in the later stages of healing, apply moisturizers (*see* p.186) to soothe the skin and prevent it from drying out.

PRACTICAL TECHNIQUE

Cooling a burn
Follow these steps to take the heat out of a burn as soon as possible. Use them for minor burns and to cool a more serious burn while you wait for help.

1 *Hold the burned area under cold running water for at least 10 minutes or until pain is relieved If water isn't available, use cold, harmless liquids such as milk or canned drinks. Do not use ice. Then pat the area dry.*

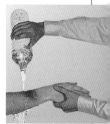

2 *Once the burn has cooled, gently remove anything that might constrict the area if it starts to swell, such as clothing, jewellery, watches, belts, or shoes.*

CAUTION: *Don't try to remove clothing or material that is stuck to burned skin. Cut around the burn and seek medical attention.*

3 *Apply cling film along the length of the arm or put a plastic bag over a burned hand or foot. Alternatively, use a sterile, non-adherent dressing or any clean, non-fluffy material, and bandage loosely. Do not put lotions or creams on a burn.*

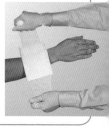

Shock

This life-threatening condition occurs when the blood circulation fails, and vital organs such as the brain and heart are deprived of oxygen. The most common cause is severe blood loss, but loss of other body fluids, as occurs in severe burns, can also cause shock. The first signs are a rapid pulse; sweating; and pale, clammy skin. These are followed by a weak pulse; rapid, shallow breathing; thirst; restlessness; and weakness. The casualty may become unconscious. If treatment is not given, the heart will stop.

> **WARNING**
>
> Call an ambulance immediately. A casualty suffering from shock needs urgent medical attention. If a casualty has a broken leg, do not raise the injured leg.

PRACTICAL TECHNIQUE

Treating signs of shock

Shock deprives the brain, heart, and other vital organs of oxygen, so the main aims of treatment are to improve the blood supply to the casualty's vital organs and to get him or her to hospital as soon as possible.

CAUTION: Stay with the casualty continually, unless you have to leave him or her in order to call an ambulance. Keep the casualty still. Do not give anything to eat or drink; if the casualty complains of feeling thirsty, moisten his or her lips with a little water.

1 *Call an ambulance. Treat any obvious cause of shock, such as severe bleeding (see p.157) or a burn (see opposite page). Be aware that there may be internal bleeding from an injury such as a major fracture. Gently help the casualty to lie down, ideally on a blanket. If his or her legs are uninjured, raise and support them on a chair or on cushions. Keeping the legs higher than the heart improves blood supply to the heart and brain. Keeping the head low may help to prevent loss of consciousness.*

Use pillows or a pile of folded coats to keep the casualty's legs raised higher than the head

Check the casualty's pulse regularly until help arrives

2 *Loosen the casualty's clothes at the neck, chest, and waist. Cover with a blanket or coat to keep him or her warm, but don't apply a direct source of heat such as a hot-water bottle. Monitor and record his or her breathing, pulse, and level of consciousness regularly. If the casualty becomes unconscious, be prepared to start CPR (see pp.170–171) if he or she stops breathing.*

Cover the casualty completely to keep him or her warm

Seizures

A seizure, also called a convulsion or fit, usually leads to a sudden partial or complete loss of consciousness. During a seizure, the person may cry out and fall, and may go rigid, with an arched back and convulsive movements. The most common cause of seizures is epilepsy, but they may also occur after a head injury, with poisoning (such as from alcohol), or with some brain disorders. In children they are often due to a high temperature; these fits are called febrile seizures (*see* opposite page).

> **WARNING**
>
> Call an ambulance if:
> ● A seizure lasts longer than 5 minutes; unconsciousness lasts longer than 10 minutes; multiple seizures occur
> ● It is a person's first seizure or you suspect head injury or poisoning

PRACTICAL TECHNIQUE

Helping during a seizure

Seizures may look alarming, but most last no longer than a few minutes and do not cause permanent damage. There is little you can do to help the casualty to regain consciousness. You can, however, protect him or her from injury; keep a regular check on the breathing, pulse, and level of response during and after the seizure; and arrange emergency help if it is needed.

1 *If you see the casualty falling, try to ease the fall by standing behind him or her. Remove any potentially dangerous items, such as hot drinks or sharp instruments, and place them out of reach. Make space around the casualty by asking bystanders to move away.*

Place a cushion or soft padding under the head

2 *If possible, protect the casualty's head by placing a cushion or soft padding underneath it. Loosen any clothing around the neck. Note the time the seizure started, so you can time how long it lasts.*

CAUTION: *Never try to restrain the casualty or put anything in the mouth.*

3 *After the seizure, the casualty may fall into a deep sleep. If breathing, put him or her into the recovery position (see p.169). Monitor and record the level of response, pulse, and breathing until he or she recovers. If breathing stops, get someone to call an ambulance and be prepared to start CPR (see pp.170–171).*

Casualty is placed in the recovery position

4 *Call an ambulance if you are unsure that the casualty is prone to epileptic seizures; if he or she is unconscious for more than 10 minutes; convulses for longer than 5 minutes; or has repeated seizures. If none of the above apply, stay with the casualty until he or she has recovered completely. Note how long the seizure lasted. Arrange for the casualty to go home and suggest that he or she seeks medical advice.*

Febrile seizures

Febrile seizures are fairly common in children, particularly between the ages of 1 and 4 years. In most cases, they are triggered by a high temperature during an illness. At first the child is hot, flushed, and sweaty, the eyes may roll upwards, and the child may arch his or her back and clench the fists. He or she may become unconscious, and there may be shaking and twitching of the limbs and body. Normally, the seizure passes quickly, but it is important to cool the child down.

> ### WARNING
> Call an ambulance if a child loses consciousness. Even if the child doesn't become fully unconscious, a doctor must see him or her as soon as possible to rule out an underlying medical condition.

PRACTICAL TECHNIQUE

Helping during a febrile seizure

Although febrile seizures often look alarming, they are unlikely to cause lasting harm to the child if they are dealt with properly and promptly. Your priorities are to protect your child from injury, to cool him or her down, and then to seek medical advice to eliminate any serious underlying causes for the seizure. If your child becomes unconscious at any time during a febrile seizure, call an ambulance.

1 *Place pillows, cushions, or soft padding around your child so that even violent movement will not result in injury. While the child is having a seizure, do not try to move him or her or put anything in the mouth.*

Put rolled-up towels on both sides of the head

2 *Undress your child down to the pants, and ensure a supply of fresh, cool air. Do not sponge a child to cool him or her.*

Gently remove clothing to cool the child

3 *Once the seizure has stopped, encourage your child to lie on his or her side and cover him or her with a light blanket or sheet. When the child wakes, you can give the recommended dose of paracetamol (see p.187) if he or she is fully conscious, but only if you are treating your own child. Seek medical advice.*

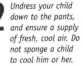

Put a light cover over the child

4 *If the child loses consciousness briefly (see p.168), call an ambulance. Put him or her in the recovery position (see p.169) and monitor and record the level of response, pulse, and breathing regularly until medical help arrives.*

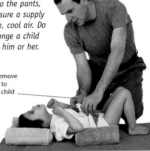

Unconsciousness

Loss of consciousness is potentially life-threatening. It has many possible causes, including a serious injury such as head injury; severe bleeding; shock; poisoning; breathing difficulty; or serious illness. An unconscious casualty will not respond to loud noises or to being tapped or shaken, and will not move or make a sound. The eyes may stay closed. If the casualty is lying face upwards, there is a risk of the tongue blocking the airway, and of choking if he or she vomits. If breathing stops, resuscitation will be needed.

WARNING

Call an ambulance.

A casualty who is unconscious needs emergency medical help.

PRACTICAL TECHNIQUE

Helping an unconscious casualty

Your priorities are to get emergency medical help and to assess the casualty's response, monitor breathing, and maintain an open airway until help arrives. It is important to prevent him or her from choking on the tongue or on any debris in the airway. If the casualty is breathing, look for and treat any obvious injuries. Be prepared to begin cardiopulmonary resuscitation (CPR) if breathing stops.

1 *Speaking loudly and clearly, ask the casualty simple questions such as "what is your name?" Tell the casualty to open the eyes. Gently shake the shoulders (tap the shoulder of a child; tap the foot of a baby). If the casualty is conscious, leave the casualty as you found him or her and check for life-threatening injuries. Call an ambulance, then treat any other obvious injuries.*

CAUTION: Always assume that the casualty has a neck injury, and handle him or her very gently.

2 *If there is no response, shout for help. Open the casualty's airway by placing one hand on the forehead, gently tilting the head back, and lifting the chin with your fingertips; the mouth will fall open slightly. Check whether the casualty is breathing, for up to 10 seconds: look for chest movement, listen for breathing sounds, and feel for breath on your cheek.*

Listen for breathing sounds

Watch the chest to detect any movement

3 *If the casualty is breathing normally, place him or her in the recovery position (see opposite page). Look for and treat any life-threatening injuries, such as bleeding (see p.157), and call an ambulance. Then treat any other obvious injuries. Monitor and record the level of response, pulse, and breathing regularly until medical help arrives.*

4 *If the casualty is not breathing normally, ask a helper to call an ambulance. Begin chest compressions and rescue breaths (see CPR, p.170). When help arrives, describe what happened and any treatment you have given.*

PRACTICAL TECHNIQUE

Recovery position (adults and children over 1 year)

If a casualty is unconscious but still breathing, place him or her in the recovery position, as shown below. This position will keep the body stable, with the head and spine aligned, and will prevent him or her from choking on the tongue or on vomit. It will also keep the airway open and clear. The technique is the same for children over 1 as for adults. (If the casualty is found lying on his or her side or front, you can adapt these steps as necessary.)

1 *Kneel beside the casualty. Remove any spectacles, and any bulky objects, such as mobile phones or keys, from his or her pockets.*

Lay the back of the hand against the face

2 *If the casualty is on his or her back, place the arm nearer to you at right angles to the body, with the elbow bent and the palm upwards. Bring the further hand across the chest and hold this hand against the cheek. Grasp the thigh further from you and pull it so that the casualty rolls towards you on to his or her side.*

Grasp the lower thigh, just behind the knee

Let the knee and foot rest on the ground

3 *Once the casualty is lying on his or her side, adjust the upper leg so that the hip and knee are bent at right angles. The knee will then support the body. Tilt the head back slightly to keep the airway open, and adjust the hand under the cheek so that the head is supported in this position.*

Recovery position (babies)

• For an unconscious but breathing baby over 1 year, open the airway, then follow the steps described above to place him or her in the recovery position.
• For an unconscious but breathing baby under 1 year, open the airway and cradle him or her in your arms with the head downwards. This position will keep the baby's airway open and allow fluids to drain from the mouth.

Hold the baby's head lower than the body

Support the lower body securely

CPR (adults)

If a casualty is unconscious and is not breathing, you need to breathe for him or her (rescue breaths) and maintain blood circulation (chest compressions). Together, these are known as cardiopulmonary resuscitation (CPR). For adults, initially it is more important to give chest compressions. However, after about 5 minutes you need to start giving rescue breaths as well.

WARNING

If you are on your own, call an ambulance before you start chest compressions unless the casualty has drowned. In this case, treat as for a child (see opposite).

PRACTICAL TECHNIQUE

CPR for adults

Use these procedures to maintain a casualty's breathing and circulation until help arrives. If you know a casualty has choked, go straight to choking (*see* p.172).

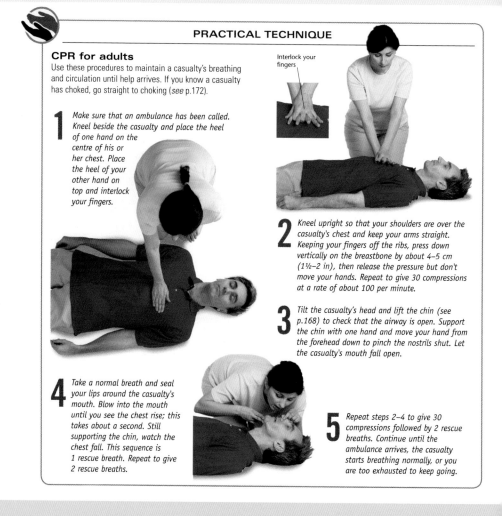

Interlock your fingers

1 Make sure that an ambulance has been called. Kneel beside the casualty and place the heel of one hand on the centre of his or her chest. Place the heel of your other hand on top and interlock your fingers.

2 Kneel upright so that your shoulders are over the casualty's chest and keep your arms straight. Keeping your fingers off the ribs, press down vertically on the breastbone by about 4–5 cm (1½–2 in), then release the pressure but don't move your hands. Repeat to give 30 compressions at a rate of about 100 per minute.

3 Tilt the casualty's head and lift the chin (see p.168) to check that the airway is open. Support the chin with one hand and move your hand from the forehead down to pinch the nostrils shut. Let the casualty's mouth fall open.

4 Take a normal breath and seal your lips around the casualty's mouth. Blow into the mouth until you see the chest rise; this takes about a second. Still supporting the chin, watch the chest fall. This sequence is 1 rescue breath. Repeat to give 2 rescue breaths.

5 Repeat steps 2–4 to give 30 compressions followed by 2 rescue breaths. Continue until the ambulance arrives, the casualty starts breathing normally, or you are too exhausted to keep going.

CPR (babies and children)

If a baby or child up to the age of puberty is unconscious and is not breathing, you need to give cardiopulmonary resuscitation (CPR), which is a combination of rescue breaths and chest compressions. For this age group, it is more likely that a breathing problem has caused the heart to stop, so you should give 5 initial rescue breaths before starting chest compressions.

WARNING
If you are on your own, give CPR for I minute before calling an ambulance.

PRACTICAL TECHNIQUE

CPR for children 1 year to puberty
This technique is for babies and children from 1 year old up to the age of puberty; for older children, see opposite.

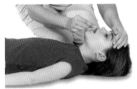

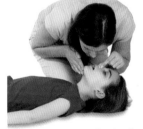

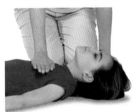

1 *If you have help, get the person to call an ambulance. Tilt and lift the child's chin (see p.168) to check that the airway is open. Remove any obvious obstructions from the mouth but do not feel for obstructions with your fingers.*

2 *Support the chin with one hand and move the hand from the forehead down to pinch the nostrils shut. Let the child's mouth fall open.*

3 *Take a normal breath and seal your lips around the child's mouth (or the mouth and nose for a baby). Blow into the mouth until you see the chest rise; this takes about a second. Still supporting the chin, watch the chest fall. This sequence is 1 rescue breath. Repeat to give 5 initial rescue breaths.*

4 *Place the heel of one hand on the centre of the child's chest, keeping your fingers off the ribcage and abdomen. Lean forward so that your shoulders are over the chest. Keeping your arms straight and your fingers off the chest, press down vertically on the breastbone by about a third of its depth, then release the pressure but don't move your hands. Repeat to give 30 compressions at a rate of about 100 per minute.*

5 *Check that the airway is open and give 2 rescue breaths. Continue the sequence of 30 compressions followed by 2 rescue breaths for 1 minute then call an ambulance if this has not already been done. Continue the sequence of 30 compressions and 2 breaths until the ambulance arrives, the child starts to breathe normally, or you are too exhausted to continue.*

CPR (babies under 1 year)
- Place your mouth over the baby's mouth and nose to give rescue breaths. Give 5 initial breaths (as above). Then place 2 fingers on the centre of the chest to give compressions. Give 30 compressions followed by 2 rescue breaths, and continue this sequence of 30 compressions and 2 breaths.

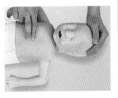

Choking

When a casualty is choking, the airway leading to the lungs is obstructed, often by a piece of food. The casualty may cough and gasp, go red in the face, have difficulty speaking, and get very distressed. Often, coughing alone is enough to clear the blockage; if it does not, first aid measures are necessary to prevent loss of consciousness. However, do not interfere while a casualty is still breathing or you may move the obstruction further down into the windpipe or lungs.

> **WARNING**
>
> Call an ambulance if:
> • The person loses consciousness
> • You cannot dislodge the blockage using the steps here
> Anybody who has had abdominal thrusts must be seen by a doctor.

PRACTICAL TECHNIQUE

Dealing with choking (adults)

Your main aim is to clear the blockage from the casualty's throat as quickly as possible.

CAUTION: Do not put your fingers in the casualty's mouth or throat in an attempt to find any trapped object. If you can see an object, pick it out with your finger and thumb.

1 *If the casualty is breathing, speaking, or coughing, encourage him or her to keep doing this. If he or she has cannot speak, breathe, or cough, give back slaps. Bend the casualty forwards and, standing behind, give 5 firm back slaps, with the flat of your hand, between the shoulderblades. Check the casualty's mouth to see if the object has been dislodged.*

Keep your hand straight when giving back slaps

Support casualty's body with your other hand

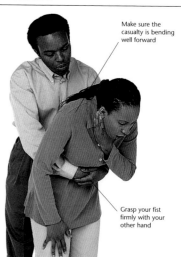

Make sure the casualty is bending well forward

Grasp your fist firmly with your other hand

2 *If back slaps fail to dislodge the blockage, try abdominal thrusts. Stand behind the casualty and put both arms around him or her. Place a clenched fist, thumb inwards, just below the ribs, between the navel and the breastbone. Grasp your fist with your other hand, and pull inwards and upwards sharply up to 5 times. Check the casualty's mouth.*

3 *If abdominal thrusts don't work, repeat the sequence of 5 back slaps followed by 5 abdominal thrusts up to 3 times or until the blockage clears. If the blockage still has not cleared, call an ambulance then continue the cycle. If the casualty becomes unconscious, get ready to perform CPR (see p.170).*

PRACTICAL TECHNIQUE

Dealing with choking (children aged 1 to puberty)

You need to clear the blockage from the throat as quickly as possible. Encourage the child to cough and do not intervene until he or she stops coughing. You may need to kneel down to use first aid techniques on a child.

1 *If the child is breathing, speaking, or coughing, encourage him or her to keep doing this. If he or she cannot breathe, speak, or cough, give back slaps. Stand or kneel behind the child and bend him or her forwards. Give up to 5 back slaps between the shoulderblades. Check the mouth and remove any obstruction you can see.*

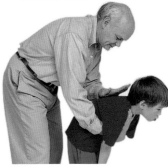

2 *If back slaps do not work, use abdominal thrusts. Place your fist against the child's upper abdomen and press sharply inwards and upwards up to 5 times.*

Fist should be just above the child's navel

3 *If abdominal thrusts don't work, repeat the sequence of 5 back slaps followed by 5 abdominal thrusts up to 3 times or until the blockage clears. If the blockage still has not cleared, call an ambulance then continue the cycle. If the child becomes unconscious, get ready to perform CPR (see p.171).*

Dealing with choking (babies under 1 year)

A choking baby may try to cry but instead make strange noises or no sound at all. If the baby cannot cry, cough, or breathe, give back slaps and, if necessary, chest thrusts.

CAUTION: Never attempt to use abdominal thrusts on a baby under 1 year old.

1 *Lay the baby face down along your forearm, supporting the body and head. Give up to 5 slaps on the baby's back with the heel of your hand. Turn the baby face up on to your other arm, check the baby's mouth and remove any visible objects.*

Make sure baby's head is below level of the chest

2 *If choking persists, place 2 fingertips on the lower half of the breastbone just below the level of the nipples. Give up to 5 downward thrusts to the chest. Check the mouth again.*

Push downwards on the breastbone with your fingertips

Support the baby's head securely

3 *If chest thrusts don't work, repeat the sequence of 5 back slaps followed by 5 chest thrusts up to 3 times or until the blockage clears. If the blockage still has not cleared, call an ambulance. If the baby becomes unconscious, get ready to perform CPR (see p.171).*

Swallowed poisons

If a poisonous substance is swallowed it can harm the mouth and digestive tract; it may also get into the bloodstream and cause further damage. Household products such as bleach, dishwasher detergent, and paint stripper contain strong chemicals that are poisonous, and many medicines are harmful if taken in excessive doses. Some plants and fungi are poisonous if eaten. The effects of poisoning vary, but there may be vomiting, a burning sensation or pain in the gullet or abdomen, and loss of consciousness.

> **WARNING**
>
> Call an ambulance.
> A casualty who has swallowed a poison or chemical needs emergency medical attention.

PRACTICAL TECHNIQUE

Dealing with swallowed poisons

The most important step is to arrange for medical help. Try to find out what poison was taken, and be ready to resuscitate if the casualty becomes unconscious or stops breathing.

CAUTION: Do not try to make the casualty vomit, as this could do further harm. If he or she has swallowed a corrosive poison, it will burn the throat again if it is vomited up.

Wipe the mouth carefully to remove traces of poison

1 Call an ambulance. Try to find out what substance was swallowed and how much. Tell the operator; these details will help the medical team decide on treatment. If the casualty can't tell you what he or she has taken, look for any empty bottles or other items that might suggest what has been consumed, and keep them to show the medical team.

2 Remove any contaminated clothing and wipe away any remaining poison from around the mouth. Take care not to get any poison on uncontaminated areas or on your own skin.

3 If the lips are burned from a corrosive chemical, give sips of cold milk or water to soothe the mouth and throat. Reassure the casualty. If alcohol poisoning is a possibility, cover the casualty with a blanket so that he or she doesn't become too cold.

Encourage the casualty to take small, frequent sips of cold milk or water

4 If the casualty becomes unconscious (see p.168), open the mouth and gently remove any substances that you can see. If breathing, put him or her in the recovery position (see p.169). Monitor and record the pulse, breathing, and level of response regularly. Be prepared to carry out CPR (see pp.170–171) if necessary. If the casualty has swallowed a corrosive substance, use a face mask when giving rescue breaths.

A-Z OF DRUG AND NATURAL REMEDIES

In this section you will find general advice on buying and using home treatments safely, and an alphabetical list of all the drugs and natural remedies that have been suggested as treatments for conditions. Each entry for a drug or remedy includes common brand names, a reminder of its most common applications, methods of use, possible side effects, and particular precautions. By necessity, only basic information can be provided here, so always refer to the full instructions supplied with the treatment, and talk to your doctor or pharmacist if you need further advice.

A–Z of drug and natural remedies

A wide range of medicines is available for home use without a doctor's prescription, as well as many herbal and other natural remedies. Using these safely is an essential part of any home treatment. In this section, you will find information on drugs and natural remedies that have been included in articles in this book, but this is only a basic guide. The advice here is not intended to replace the guidance of medical professionals, so always consult a doctor or pharmacist if you need more information. It is also essential that you read and follow the instructions provided with any drug or remedy and pay particular attention to cautions.

How to use this section

Drugs and natural remedies are listed here alphabetically, and there are cross references to them from the articles in which they are mentioned. Natural remedies are indicated by a leaf symbol and drug entries by a tablet symbol.

At the beginning of each drug entry there is a list of selected common brands with the main ingredients of each brand given in brackets. Where a drug has several applications, the brands for different uses are shown.

Some basic instructions on method of use are provided, but details may vary from one product to another, so always refer to information supplied with the product. Common side effects, if any, are given. Under precautions, you will find concerns that apply when using the product, specific circumstances in which it should not be used, and a cross reference to the GENERAL CAUTIONS (below) when applicable.

General cautions

Although many of the medicines included here can be used safely for most people most of the time, there are situations when extra care is needed or when some treatments should be avoided altogether. Listed below are general cautions that apply when taking medicines and natural remedies. You should also read and follow the instructions and cautions included with the product.

● If you are pregnant or breastfeeding, consult a doctor or pharmacist before using any drug or remedy.

● Speak to your doctor or pharmacist before using a medicine if you have liver or kidney problems or any other long-term medical condition, such as a stomach ulcer, diabetes, heart disease, or high blood pressure. Drugs and remedies may have stronger or different effects because of a chronic illness.

● Before treating babies and children, make sure you are certain of the diagnosis and the suitability of the medicine. Check dosages for different age ranges. Consult your doctor or pharmacist first if you are in doubt about the treatment.

● If you are already taking prescribed medication, talk to your doctor before taking a new drug or remedy. Over-the-counter drugs and natural remedies can interact with each other and with prescribed medicines, sometimes with potentially harmful results. However, don't stop taking prescribed medicine without first consulting your doctor.

● Store medicines and remedies in a cool, dry place, out of reach of children. Check use-by dates and dispose of any medicines and remedies that are out of date.

Using natural remedies safely

Although there is a huge variety of natural remedies available in pharmacies and health stores, only a small number appear in this book. Those that have been included have been selected on the basis that they have undergone medical testing and there is some evidence of their safety and effectiveness. The few exceptions are herbal teas and sleep remedies that may help and are unlikely to cause harm.

A concern when using natural remedies is that much of the evidence for them is anecdotal, and testing of them is usually less rigorous than for conventional drugs. In addition, quality and dosages are not regulated or standardized, so there is no guarantee of their strength, purity, and safety, and their effects cannot be predicted exactly. When buying natural remedies, always use a reputable supplier and make sure there are full instructions and warnings with the product. Observe these carefully and don't exceed the recommended dose.

When taking any remedy, be aware that although many of them are derived from plants and have the label "natural" or "herbal", they are not natural to the human body and can have effects that are as strong as those of conventional drugs. Natural remedies can also interact with other drugs and substances, such as alcohol. Cautions also apply in the same circumstances as conventional drugs (*see* GENERAL CAUTIONS, left).

Aciclovir cream

Common brands
● Herpetad ● Soothelip ● Zovirax cream

Antiviral drug that attacks the herpes cold-sore virus, reducing the duration and severity of cold sores.

Method of use Most effective if used at first sign of tingling. Apply a thin layer.

Side effects Occasionally, mild stinging or burning initially; skin may be irritated, red, or dry.

Precautions Wash hands before and after use. Don't use near eyes or inside the mouth or vagina; if the drug gets in an eye, rinse well; if stinging occurs, consult a doctor.

Aloe vera

The aloe plant (*Aloe vera*) is a centuries-old remedy for skin conditions such as sunburn and psoriasis. May help relieve pain and swelling and speed healing.

Method of use Available in skin creams, gels, and ointments. Apply as needed.

Side effects Usually none.

Precautions None.

Aluminium chloride

Common brands
● Anhydrol Forte ● Driclor

Controls severe or excessive sweating by blocking sweat ducts; use when other methods do not help.

Method of use Available as sprays and roll-on applicators. Apply to clean, dry skin before going to bed; wash off the next morning.

Side effects Possible skin irritation.

Precautions Use only on small areas, such as palms or armpits. Don't use on shaved, irritated, or broken skin, or near eyes or lips. Don't use depilatories 12 hours before or after treatment. Keep away from fabrics, jewellery, metal, and polished objects.

Antacids

Common brands
MIXTURES OF CHEMICAL COMPOUNDS: ● Bisodol Indigestion Relief Tablets (calcium, magnesium, sodium bicarbonate) ● Phillips' Milk of Magnesia (magnesium) ● Remegel (calcium) ● Rennie (calcium, magnesium) ● Setlers Antacid (calcium) WITH DIMETICONE: ● Asilone Antacid Liquid (aluminium, dimeticone, magnesium) ● Maalox Plus Suspension (aluminium, magnesium, dimeticone)

WITH ALGINATES: ● Gaviscon Advance (alginic acid, potassium bicarbonate, calcium carbonate)

Contain various compounds that relieve indigestion and heartburn by neutralizing stomach acid. Some also contain dimeticone (also called simethicone) to absorb excess stomach gas. Others contain alginates that help prevent acid reflux, which causes heartburn.

Method of use Available as hard or chewy tablets, fizzy drinks, or soothing liquids. Method of use varies; follow instructions on packet.

Side effects Usually none.

Precautions Antacids can interfere with absorption of some drugs; check with a doctor or pharmacist before use if already taking other medicines. *See also* GENERAL CAUTIONS, opposite page.

Anti-dandruff shampoos

Common brands
● Capasal (coal tar, salicylic acid) ● Neutrogena T/Gel (coal tar) ● Nizoral Dandruff Shampoo (ketoconazole) ● Polytar AF (coal tar, pyrithione zinc) ● Selsun (selenium sulphide)

Selenium sulphide and pyrithione zinc shampoos reduce overgrowth of a type of fungus living on the scalp, a common cause of dandruff. Ketoconazole, an antifungal drug, is very effective, often when other treatments don't work. Coal tar shampoos (*see also* p.179), alone or with salicylic acid, reduce scaling and can also be used to treat cradle cap in babies.

Method of use As directed. Beneficial effect may not be apparent for a few weeks.

Side effects Occasionally, itching, irritation, or burning sensation on the scalp.

Precautions Avoid eyes and inflamed or broken skin. Coal tar shampoos may stain blonde or grey hair; may also increase the risk of sunburn for up to 24 hours; protect your head from strong sunshine. *See also* GENERAL CAUTIONS, opposite page.

Antidiarrhoeal drugs

Common brands
● Boots Diareze Diarrhoea Relief (loperamide) ● Diocalm Ultra (loperamide) ● Imodium (loperamide)

Diarrhoea is best left to run its course, but when essential, medicines may be taken as a short-term measure to slow bowel activity.

Method of use Use as needed. Take the lowest dose that helps. Drink plenty of clear fluids to prevent dehydration.

Side effects Usually none; constipation, nausea, tiredness, dry mouth, or a rash may occur.

Precautions *See* GENERAL CAUTIONS, p.176.

Antifungal drugs

Common brands
RINGWORM: ● Canesten (clotrimazole)
● Daktarin (miconazole)
ATHLETE'S FOOT: ● Canesten AF (clotrimazole)
● Daktarin Dual Action (miconazole)
● Lamisil AT (terbinafine)
VAGINAL THRUSH: ● Canesten Cream (clotrimazole)
● Canesten Oral Capsule (fluconazole) ● Canesten Duo (clotrimazole cream and fluconazole tablet)

Treat fungal conditions, such as ringworm, athlete's foot, or vaginal thrush.

Method of use Cream, powder, or spray powder for skin infections. As pessaries, cream (with applicator), a fluconazole capsule (taken orally), or a combination clotrimazole (cream) and fluconazole (oral tablet) for vaginal thrush. Wash hands after use.

Side effects Occasionally, irritation and redness; if severe, stop using and consult a doctor. Fluconazole may cause nausea, abdominal pain, wind, and diarrhoea.

Precautions For topical products, avoid eyes, nose, mouth, or broken or sensitive skin. Vaginal pessaries and creams may damage latex condoms and diaphragms. *See also* GENERAL CAUTIONS, p.176.

Antihistamines

Common brands
NON-SEDATING: ● Benadryl One a Day Relief (cetirizine) ● Clarityn Allergy (loratadine)
SEDATING: ● Nytol (diphenhydramine) ● Phenergan (promethazine) ● Piriton (chlorphenamine)
CREAM: ● Anthisan (mepyramine)
EYE DROPS: ● Otrivine-Antistin (antazoline, xylometazoline)

Control allergic symptoms such as sneezing and runny nose. Also itchy eyes, and itchy and inflamed skin from insect bites or nettle rash. Sedative types can be used as a short-term sleeping aid.

Method of use Tablets and liquids taken as soon as allergic reaction occurs, or to prevent one. Use eye drops 2–3 times a day. Apply creams thinly to bites or stings.

Side effects Sedating types may cause drowsiness for a few days. Non-sedating types less so, but caution needed.

Precautions Don't take sedating types if driving or operating hazardous machinery. Don't use eye drops if you wear contact lenses or have glaucoma. *See also* GENERAL CAUTIONS, p.176.

Anti-nailbiting lotions

Common brands
● Mavala Stop ● Stop'n Grow

Help stop nailbiting. Contain bitter-tasting, but harmless, chemicals.

Method of use Apply directly to nail surfaces. Use every day.

Side effects Usually none.

Precautions Don't use on broken or sensitive skin, and avoid eyes and lips. Check instructions before use on children.

Antispasmodic drugs

Common brands
● Buscopan IBS Relief (hyoscine) ● Colofac IBS (mebeverine) ● Colpermin (peppermint oil)
● Relaxyl (alverine)

Help to relax the bowel muscle and relieve pain and bloating in irritable bowel syndrome.

Method of use Tablets or capsules.

Side effects Peppermint oil may cause heartburn; alverine may cause nausea, headache, dizziness, and a rash; mebeverine may, rarely, trigger an allergic skin reaction; hyoscine may cause dry mouth, problems with urination, or vision problems, such as burred vision.

Precautions Not recommended for children. Hyoscine should not be used by those with glaucoma. It may also interact with other drugs; check with you pharmacist first if you are taking other medications. *See also* GENERAL CAUTIONS, p.176.

Aromatic oils

Eucalyptus, camphor, and menthol used for treating colds and blocked sinuses. Inhaling vapours helps unblock the nose and ease breathing.

Method of use Oils, chest rubs, and lozenges. Inhale a few drops of oil placed on a tissue; at bedtime, place tissue inside the pillowcase. Apply a rub to the chest, throat, and back. Suck menthol lozenges to relieve a stuffed-up nose.

Side effects Usually none.

Precautions None.

Aspirin

Common brands:
- Alka-Seltzer ● Anadin Extra Soluble Tablets
- Anadin Original ● Aspro Clear ● Disprin

Relieves mild to moderate pain in conditions such as migraine, sore throat, toothache, and joint pain and inflammation. Reduces fever. Included in medicines for colds, flu, period pains, and joint and muscle aches.

Method of use Coated, regular, or soluble (fastest acting) tablets. Take with or after food.

Side effects Indigestion due to irritation of the stomach lining; less likely with coated tablets.

Precautions Consult a doctor first if you have or have had asthma or a stomach disorder. Don't use if you are allergic to aspirin or other anti-inflammatory drugs. *See also* GENERAL CAUTIONS, p.176.

 WARNING
Don't give aspirin to child under 16, unless on doctor's advice. There is a risk of a rare, but potentially fatal, condition called Reye's syndrome.

Benzoyl peroxide

Common brands
- Acnecide ● Brevoxyl ● PanOxyl

Preparations for mild or moderate acne reduce inflammation and bacteria and make skin less oily.

Method of use Available as gels, lotions, or creams. Wash skin first. Start with low strength; move on to a higher strength only if needed.

Side effects Skin may redden, peel, and become dry and irritated, but this normally resolves in a few days if treatment is stopped temporarily; if not, use less frequently; if severe, stop using.

Precautions Don't apply to damaged skin. Avoid eyes, lips, mouth, and lining of nose. Benzoyl peroxide can bleach hair and clothes.

Calamine lotion

Common brands
- Boots Calamine and Glycerin Cream
- Calamine Lotion

Has a cooling effect and is used to soothe minor skin irritation and rashes.

Method of use Available as lotion or cream. Apply as often as needed. Dab lotion on to skin with cotton wool and leave to dry.

Side effects Usually none.

Precautions Usually none.

Calendula cream

 Creams prepared from extracts of marigold, or calendula (*Calendula officinalis*), traditionally used to soothe cuts, grazes, and mild skin inflammation.

Method of use Available in creams or lotions. Apply as directed on packet.

Side effects *See* GENERAL CAUTIONS, p.176.

Precautions Usually none.

Chloramphenicol

Common brand:
- Optrex Infected Eyes (eye drops, ointment)

Used to treat bacterial conjunctivitis.

Method of use Wash hands before use. Apply inside lower eyelid. Keep droppers or nozzles away from eyeball or any other surfaces.

Side effects Brief stinging or blurred vision.

Precautions Not for use in children under 2 years. Consult a doctor if symptoms do not improve within 48 hours. *See also* GENERAL CAUTIONS, p.176.

Coal tar preparations

Common brands
CREAMS AND LOTIONS: ● Clinitar ● Exorex ● Psoriderm ● Cocois (with salicylic acid)
SHAMPOOS: ●Polytar AF ●Capasal (with salicylic acid)
BATH ADDITIVES: ● Polytar Emollient ● Psoriderm

Used in conditions such as psoriasis to reduce inflammation and scaling. Available as a cream, paste, lotion, shampoo (*see also* ANTI-DANDRUFF SHAMPOOS, p.177), or bath additive. Coal tar with salicylic acid is used to treat scalp psoriasis.

Method of use Apply cream, paste, or lotion to clean skin. Wash hands after use. Add bath products to a warm bath. Use shampoos as directed.

Side effects Coal tar can irritate skin or cause a rash. If this occurs, stop using.

Precautions Don't use on broken skin or inflamed or infected psoriasis. Avoid eyes and lining of nose and mouth. Avoid exposing skin to sunlight.

Cold and flu remedies

Common brands
- Beechams All in One (guaifenesin, paracetamol, phenylephrine) ● Lemsip Cold and Flu Lemon (paracetamol, phenylephrine, vitamin C) ● Lemsip Cold & Flu Max Strength Capsules (paracetamol, phenylephrine, caffeine)

● Non-Drowsy Sudafed Dual Relief (paracetamol, phenylephrine, caffeine) ● Nurofen Cold and Flu (ibuprofen, pseudoephedrine)

Help relieve headache, fever, sore throat, cough, and blocked nose or sinuses. May contain a painkiller, such as paracetamol (*see* p.187), which also helps to reduce fever; a decongestant, such as phenylephrine (*see* p.180), to help unblock nose and sinuses; an antihistamine, such as pseudoephedrine (*see* opposite page), for a runny nose; cough suppressants (*see* p.180); and expectorants, such as guaifenesin.

Method of use Available as tablets, liquid, or soluble powders.

Side effects See entries for ingredients.

Precautions *See* GENERAL CAUTIONS, p.176.

 WARNING
Don't take remedies containing painkillers with other painkillers due to risk of overdose. Don't take remedies containing decongestants if you have taken MAOI antidepressants in the last 14 days. Remedies containing aspirin must not be given to a child under 16, except on a doctor's advice.

Cough suppressants

 Common brands
● Benylin Dry Cough (dextromethorphan, diphenhydramine, menthol) ● Night Nurse (dextromethorphan, paracetamol, promethazine) ● Boots Nirolex Dry Cough and Congestion Relief Linctus (dextromethorphan, pseudoephedrine) ● Boots Nirolex Night Time Cough Relief Linctus (diphenhydramine, pholcodine)

Pholcodine or dextromethorphan remedies for a dry, irritating cough, not for coughs that produce mucus. Suppressants may also contain sedating antihistamines, such as diphenhydramine and promethazine (*see* p.178); painkillers, such as paracetamol (*see* p.187); and decongestants, such as pseudoephedrine (*see* right).

Method of use Usually liquids. Take as directed; for coughing at night, take at bedtime.

Side effects Antihistamines may cause drowsiness, dizziness, dry mouth, blurred vision, or difficulty urinating. Dextromethorphan may cause dizziness, nausea, or stomach upsets. Pholcodine may cause constipation.

Precautions Don't take with alcohol. If drowsy, don't drive or use hazardous machinery. Consult doctor before use if you have glaucoma, or prostate, kidney, or liver problems. *See also* GENERAL CAUTIONS, p.176.

 WARNING
Don't use mixtures containing painkillers with other drugs such as paracetamol, due to risk of overdose. Don't take remedies containing decongestants if you have taken MAOI antidepressants in the last 14 days.

Counter-irritants

 Common brands
COOLING ● Deep Freeze Cold Gel (menthol) ● Ralgex Freeze Spray (dimethyl ether, glycol monosalicylate, isopentane)
WARMING ● Deep Heat Rub (eucalyptus oil, menthol, methyl salicylate, turpentine oil) ● PR Heat Spray (ethyl niconate, methyl salicate, camphor)

Produce a mild tingling in the skin to soothe pain and stiffness in muscles and joints temporarily. Some products warm and increase blood flow to the area; others have a cooling effect.

Method of use Massage cream or apply spray to the affected area. Wash hands after use.

Side effects Occasionally, irritated or reddened skin; if affected, stop using.

Precautions Avoid eyes and sensitive or broken skin. *See also* GENERAL CAUTIONS, p.176.

Crotamiton preparations

 Common brand
● Eurax cream/lotion

Relieve itching in skin problems such as hives, insect bites and stings, and after scabies treatment.

Method of use For itching, apply to affected area; for scabies, apply to whole body.

Side effects Occasionally, skin irritation or allergic reaction may occur; if affected, stop using.

Precautions Avoid eyes and broken or weeping skin. *See also* GENERAL CAUTIONS, p.176.

Cystitis relief

Common brands
● Canesten Oasis (sodium citrate) ● Cymalon (sodium citrate) ● Cystopurin Cranberry Sachets (potassium citrate)

Contain potassium citrate or sodium citrate. Make urine less acidic and reduce burning and stinging.

Method of use Take as soon as symptoms start. Dissolve contents of sachet or granules in water; drink immediately. Take the whole course (usually 2 days).

Side effects Usually none.

Precautions Consult your doctor first if you have diabetes, high blood pressure, or heart or kidney problems. *See also* GENERAL CAUTIONS, p.176.

Decongestants

Common brands
● Non-Drowsy Sudafed Decongestant Nasal Spray (xylometazoline) ● Otrivine Adult Menthol Nasal Spray (xylometazoline) ● Sudafed Decongestant tablets/elixir (pseudoephedrine) ● Vicks Sinex (oxymetazoline)

Fast-acting sprays or drops to help relieve symptoms of colds, sinusitis, and hay fever for up to 10 hours. Also available as tablets and in cold and flu remedies.

Method of use Apply drops or spray directly into each nostril; with spray, sniff as vapour is released. Take tablets or elixir orally.

Side effects Occasionally, stinging, itching, or sneezing may occur.

Precautions Don't use sprays or drops continuously for more than 7 days. Consult a doctor if you are taking prescribed drugs or have diabetes, heart disease, or high blood pressure.

 WARNING
Don't take decongestants if you have taken MAOI antidepressants in the last 14 days. *See also* GENERAL CAUTIONS, p.176.

Ear wax drops

Common brands
WAX SOFTENERS: ● Almond oil ● Olive oil ● Sodium bicarbonate ear drops
WAX SOLVENTS: ● Exterol (urea–hydrogen peroxide) ● Otex (urea–hydrogen peroxide) ● Waxsol (docusate sodium)

Softeners are effective, cheap, and usually less irritating than wax solvents.

Method of use Tilt head and apply drops into ear. Treat one ear at a time, a few days apart.

Side effects Solvents may cause brief "bubbling", mild stinging, and irritation in the ear.

Precautions Don't use if there is pain, inflammation, or damage in the ear, a burst eardrum, dizziness, or recurrent ear problems.

Echinacea

Herbal remedy believed to help the body fight infections. Used at the start of a cold, may help to reduce symptoms and speed recovery.

Method of use Available as capsules, tea, juice, or a tincture to be diluted.

Side effects Uncommon; the most likely problems are stomach upset and nausea.

Precautions Don't use for more than 8 weeks; may harm the liver. *See also* GENERAL CAUTIONS, p.176.

Emollient bath additives

Common brands
● E45 (cetyl dimeticone, liquid paraffin) ● Oilatum (acetylated wool alcohols, liquid paraffin)

Soothes dry, itchy skin in conditions such as eczema and psoriasis. May be used with aqueous creams or emollients (*see* MOISTURIZERS, p.186). Some brands contain oatmeal (*see* OATMEAL PRODUCTS, p.186).

Method of use Add to a lukewarm bath, or apply to wet skin. Pat skin dry.

Side effects Usually none.

Precautions Oils can make the bath slippery, so take care when getting in and out.

Essential fatty acids

Essential fatty acids (EFAs), particularly omega-3 EFAs, help to form cells and nerve tissue. They may also help relieve depression and period pains.

Method of use Found in foods, principally oily fish such as sardines and salmon; olive oil; walnuts; and flax seeds.

Side effects Usually none if EFAs are eaten as part of a balanced diet.

Precautions None.

Eye lubricants

Common brands
EYE DROPS: ● Isopto Plain (hypromellose) ● Tears Naturale (hypromellose) ● Sodium chloride drops
GELS: ● GelTears (carbomers) ● Viscotears (carbomers)
OINTMENT: ● Lacri-lube (liquid paraffin)

Drops and gels keep eyes moist and relieve itching and dryness. Ointment containing liquid paraffin lubricates eyes at night. Sodium chloride drops suitable for contact lens wearers.

Method of use Always wash hands before use. Apply inside lower eyelid. Keep droppers or nozzles away from eyeball or any other surfaces.

Side effects Brief stinging or blurred vision.

Precautions If vision is blurred, don't drive or use hazardous machinery. Some eye drops contain chemicals that can damage contact lenses; never wear contact lenses when using ointment. Don't use ointment in daytime as it may blur vision.

Feverfew

Feverfew (*Tanacetum parthenium*) is a garden herb found by some people to reduce the frequency and severity of migraine attacks.

Method of use Available as capsules, tablets, leaf powder, or tea.

Side effects Usually none; most likely problems are mouth inflammation or ulcers. If taken for long periods and stopped suddenly, "rebound" headaches, anxiety, and palpitations may occur.

Precautions Don't take if you are pregnant (may cause miscarriage) or breastfeeding. Avoid if taking blood-thinning drugs such as warfarin, or antidepressants. *See also* GENERAL CAUTIONS, p.176.

Flatulence relief

Common brands
● Actonorm Gel (aluminium, magnesium, dimeticone, peppermint oil) ● Asilone Antacid Liquid (aluminium, magnesium, dimeticone) ● Bisodol Wind Relief Tablets (calcium, magnesium, sodium bicarbonate, dimeticone) ● J.L. Bragg's Medicinal Charcoal Tablets (charcoal) ● Remegel Wind Relief (calcium, dimeticone) ● Rennie Deflatine (calcium, magnesium, dimeticone) ● Setlers Wind-eze (dimeticone)

Dimeticone (simethicone) breaks down bubbles of gas in stomach. Usually combined with an antacid (*see* p.177) in preparations to treat indigestion. Charcoal tablets and biscuits bind with excess gas so it can be passed out of the body.

Method of use As directed on packet. Chew or swallow charcoal tablets with a drink.

Side effects Usually none.

Precautions Charcoal tablets not recommended for children under 12.

Ginger

Common spice and flavouring. Ginger (*Zingiber officinale*) may also help to prevent or relieve nausea in conditions such as travel sickness.

Method of use Available as capsules, sweets, or tea. Can be eaten fresh, crystallized, or powdered in fruit juice. To help prevent travel sickness, take ginger 30 minutes before journey.

Side effects Brief heartburn or wind.

Precautions Not advised if you are pregnant. Check whether the product is suitable before giving to a child. *See also* GENERAL CAUTIONS, p.176.

Glucosamine and chondroitin

In arthritis, supplements of either substance or both may help to relieve pain, improve flexibility, and slow rate of damage.

Method of use Usually taken as tablets. Full effects may take at least a month; if no improvement after 10 weeks, stop using.

Side effects Usually none.

Precautions Don't take glucosamine if you are allergic to shellfish. Consult a doctor before use with blood-thinning drugs such as warfarin, or if you have diabetes. *See also* GENERAL CAUTIONS, p.176.

H2-blockers

Common brands
● Pepcidtwo (famotidine, magnesium hydroxide, calcium carbonate) ● Zantac 75 relief (ranitidine)

Reduce amounts of stomach acid to relieve occasional bouts of indigestion and heartburn. Some products contain an H2-blocker and an antacid (*see* p.177).

Method of use Effervescent tablets or chewable tablets. Recommended only for short-term use (normally no more than 2 weeks of continual use).

Side effects Usually none; most likely problems are headaches, dizziness, stomach upsets, rash, and tiredness.

Precautions Not usually recommended for children under 16. *See also* precautions for antacids (p.177) and GENERAL CAUTIONS, p.176.

Haemorrhoid preparations

Common brands:
● Anodesyn ointment/suppositories (allantoin, lidocaine) ●Anusol cream (bismuth oxide, Peru balsam, zinc oxide) ●Anusol ointment/suppositories (bismuth oxide, bismuth subgallate, Peru balsam, zinc oxide) ●Anusol Plus HC (benzyl benzoate, bismuth oxide, bismuth subgallate, hydrocortisone, Peru balsam, zinc oxide) ●Germoloids (lidocaine, zinc oxide)

Relieve anal pain, itching, and swelling. Many contain zinc oxide, a mild antiseptic; others combine zinc oxide and local anaesthetics, such as lidocaine or benzocaine, to help relieve irritation. Some contain hydrocortisone to reduce inflammation. Creams also lubricate the area, making it easier to pass stools.

Method of use Available as cream, ointment, or suppositories. Clean and dry anal area before use. Wash hands before and after use.

Side effects May sting as they are applied.

Precautions Don't use for more than 6–7 days, as may irritate anal skin; if haemorrhoids persist, consult a doctor. Some brands are unsuitable for children.

Hair bleaches

Common brand
● Jolen Creme Bleach (hydrogen peroxide)

Mild bleach used to lighten facial or body hair and make it less noticeable against fair skin.

Method of use Usually a cream supplied with ammonia to activate bleach. Mix and apply with a spatula. Use as directed on the packet.

Side effects Irritation or allergic reaction may occur; test on a small area of skin. Wait for 24 hours to make sure there is no reaction.

Precautions Don't use on broken or inflamed skin or near the eyes. Don't use just after having a bath, as the skin is sensitive, or expose treated areas to sunlight for 24 hours. Can stain clothing and furniture.

Hair removal products

Common brands
● Boots products (wax, cream) ● Nads products (wax, gel, cream) ● Nair products (wax, gel, cream, spray mousse) ● Veet products (wax, cream)

Creams, gels, and mousses dissolve hair down to the roots. Wax preparations pull out hairs, so effect lasts for a couple of weeks.

Method of use Creams and gels applied with a spatula. Mousses sprayed on and then washed off. Waxes applied to clean, dry skin with hairs at least 5 mm (¼ in) long; fabric strips applied and pulled off against the direction of hair growth.

Side effects Creams, gels, and mousses may cause irritation; if so, wash off immediately. Waxes may produce raised, red spots briefly.

Precautions Can cause allergic reactions; test on small area first. Don't use on skin that is irritated, broken, spotty, or sunburned. Don't use on moles or warts, within 2 hours of bathing or sunbathing, or within 72 hours of shaving. Wait 24 hours before using deodorants or perfumes. Avoid waxes if you have diabetes.

Hangover remedies

Common brands
● Alka-Seltzer XS (aspirin, paracetamol, caffeine, sodium carbonate, citric acid) ● Resolve Extra (paracetamol, sodium bicarbonate, caffeine)

Relieve headaches and upset stomach. Most contain combinations of drugs, including aspirin (*see* p.187) and/or paracetamol (*see* p.187) for headaches, and antacids (*see* p.178) for upset stomach. May also contain vitamin C, glucose, or caffeine.

Method of use Usually, soluble tablets or powder to be mixed with water as a drink.

Side effects Aspirin may irritate stomach.

Precautions See precautions for paracetamol and aspirin, and also GENERAL CAUTIONS, p.176.

WARNING
Don't take with painkillers due to risk of overdose. Don't give aspirin to anyone under 16, unless advised by a doctor.

Herbal sleeping remedies

Herbs such as valerian (*Valeriana officinalis*), hops (*Humulus lupulus*), passionflower (*Passiflora incarnata*), and camomile are said to aid relaxation and sleep.

Method of use Available as tablets or liquid, taken at bedtime. Camomile can be drunk as tea. Pillows stuffed with dried hops also available. Try tablets and liquids for only a few days at a time. If sleeping problem persists, consult a doctor.

Side effects Usually none.

Precautions None.

Herbal teas

Peppermint, camomile, gentian, or fennel teas traditionally used to relieve indigestion, heartburn, or wind; ginger tea (*see* p.182) used for nausea and travel sickness; camomile tea for insomnia (*see* HERBAL SLEEPING REMEDIES, above).

Method of use Add boiling water to tea, and leave to brew for a few minutes. Don't add milk.

Side effects Usually none.

Precautions Don't take ginger in pregnancy.

Hydrocolloid plasters

Common brands
CORNS, CALLUSES: ● Compeed Callus and Corn Plasters
BLISTERS: ● Boots Hydrocolloid Blister Plaster
● Compeed Blister Hydrocolloid

Dressings for corns, calluses, and blisters. Contain a substance that absorbs moisture to form a gel that cushions and protects the area. Types for corns and calluses also soften hardened skin to aid removal. Blister dressings keep skin moist and relieve pressure.

Method of use Choose plaster that covers whole area. Leave it on until it comes off by itself.

Side effects Usually none.

Precautions None.

Hydrocortisone cream

Common brands
- Hc45 ● Lanacort

Mild steroid cream reduces inflammation in non-infectious conditions, such as eczema, insect stings, and skin reactions to jewellery, plants, and toiletries. Also in some haemorrhoid preparations (*see* p.182).

Method of use Apply thinly as directed on packet. Don't put dressings over treated area.

Side effects Usually none.

Precautions Don't use for longer than a week. Don't use on the face, genital area, or broken or infected skin. Don't use on children under 10, unless on doctor's advice. See also GENERAL CAUTIONS, p.176.

Ibuprofen

Common brands
TABLETS: ● Anadin Ibuprofen ● Hedex Ibuprofen ● Nurofen
GELS: ● Ibugel ● Ibuleve
LIQUID: ● Nurofen for Children

Belongs to a group of medicines known as non-steroidal anti-inflammatory drugs (NSAIDs). Widely used to treat muscle and joint pains, headaches, cold and flu symptoms (and fever), and period pains.

Method of use Usually, tablets. Liquid for children (normally 3 months and weighing over 5kg–12 years). Take after food to minimize stomach irritation. Creams, gels, or sprays for sprains and muscular aches are applied to skin.

Side effects Usually mild; most likely problems are nausea and indigestion from tablets.

Precautions Avoid using creams or gels on or near broken skin, eyes, or mouth. Consult a doctor before using ibuprofen if you have or have had a peptic ulcer or asthma. Don't take if you have had an allergic reaction to ibuprofen, aspirin, or similar drugs, or a worsening of asthma or allergic symptoms. *See also* GENERAL CAUTIONS, p.176.

Insect bite and sting relief

Common brands
- Anthisan Bite and Sting Cream (mepyramine)
- Wasp-Eze Spray (mepyramine, benzocaine)

Most contain an antihistamine (*see* p.178), such as mepyramine, to ease swelling and itching and a local anaesthetic, such as benzocaine. Can also relieve nettle or jellyfish stings. Hydrocortisone cream (*see* left) can be used for bites and stings.

Method of use Available as creams, ointments, or sprays. Apply sparingly straight away.

Side effects Usually none. If rash occurs, stop using.

Precautions Don't apply to large areas, or to broken or sunburnt skin.

Lactase supplements

Common brands
- BioCare Lactase Enzyme (liquid) ● Quest Lactase Tablets ● Solgar Lactase 3500 (wafer)

May help people to overcome intolerance to milk or dairy products. Lactase helps to break down lactose sugar in the body so that it can be easily absorbed.

Method of use Take tablets or wafers with or just before eating or drinking dairy products. Add liquid to milk or milk products.

Side effects Usually none.

Precautions See a doctor before use if you are diabetic or think a child has a food intolerance.

Lanolin ointment

Common brand
- Lansinoh

Creams containing lanolin protect skin and soothe and heal sore and cracked nipples in breastfeeding women. Use only medical-grade lanolin products.

Method of use Apply to nipples. Does not have to be wiped off before feeding baby.

Side effects Usually none.

Precautions None.

Lavender

Lavender (*Lavendula augustifolia*) is a traditional remedy that may help some people to sleep.

Method of use Add lavender oil to a warm bath or put drops on a tissue or handkerchief and inhale. Place sachets of dried lavender inside a pillowcase to aid sleep.

Side effects Occasionally, skin irritation, nausea, and headache.

Precautions Don't use lavender oil if you are pregnant or breastfeeding.

Laxatives

Common brands
FIBRE SUPPLEMENTS: ● Celevac (methylcellulose) ● Fybogel Orange/Lemon (isphagula) ● Regulan (isphagula) ● Bran
STIMULANT LAXATIVES: ● Dulco-lax (bisacodyl) ● Ex-Lax Senna Chocolate Laxatives (senna) ● Senokot (senna)

Laxatives relieve constipation. Fibre supplements help stools retain water, making them softer, bulkier, and easier to pass. Stimulant types make bowel muscles contract and speed the passage of faeces.

Method of use Fibre supplements as granules or powder, to be mixed with water and drunk; avoid taking at bedtime. Stimulant types available as tablets, powder, syrup, or suppositories, normally taken at bedtime as they work overnight.

Side effects Mild bloating and flatulence with fibres supplements; mild abdominal discomfort just after taking stimulant types.

Precautions Drink plenty of fluids with fibre supplements. Don't use stimulant laxatives for more than 7 days at a time. Overuse may make bowels ineffective without them. Don't use if you have another digestive disorder. *See also* GENERAL CAUTIONS, p.176.

Lip creams, balms, and salves

Common brands
● Chapstick ● Lypsyl Original Lipsalve ● Piz Buin Sun Lipstick ● Vaseline Lip Therapy

Moisturize and soothe sore, chapped, and cracked lips and mouth. Petroleum-based products protect against dryness in cold weather. Ski protection types have a sun protection factor (SPF) of 15 or higher for use at high altitudes.

Method of use Available as solid sticks, creams, ointments, or gels. Apply as needed.

Side effects Usually none.

Precautions Don't use on broken skin.

Lubricating jelly

Common brands
LUBRICANTS: ●Durex Sensilube ●K–Y Lubricating Jelly
VAGINAL MOISTURIZER: ● Replens MD

Water-soluble lubricants applied to penis or vagina to ease dryness and soreness. Available as gels or vaginal moisturizers. Safe to use with condoms (unlike oil-based lubricants, which can break down latex).

Method of use Apply to vaginal entrance or penis prior to intercourse; longer-lasting vaginal moisturizers applied internally several times a week to provide continuous moisture.

Side effects Usually none.

Precautions Don't use vaginal moisturizers during or just after pregnancy.

Migraine remedies

Common brands
PAINKILLERS WITH ANTI-NAUSEA DRUG ● Migraleve (paracetamol, codeine, buclizine)
ANTI-NAUSEA DRUG ● Buccastem M (prochlorperazine)

Migraleve contains paracetamol and codeine (*see* p.187) and an anti-nausea drug to help relieve headache, nausea, and vomiting. Prochlorperazine relieves nausea for up to 12 hours.

Method of use Take Migraleve tablet at first sign of attack; may prevent migraine developing. Place prochlorperazine tablet between gum and upper lip and allow to dissolve. Use with a painkiller.

Side effects Migraleve may cause drowsiness and/or constipation. Prochlorperazine may cause drowsiness, dizziness, dry mouth, insomnia, and irritation of the gums.

Precautions Don't take with alcohol. Don't give to children under 10 except on medical advice. Don't give prochlorperazine to anyone under 18 or use for longer than 2 days. If drowsy, don't drive or operate machinery. *See also* GENERAL CAUTIONS, p.176.

 WARNING
Don't take remedies containing painkillers with other painkillers due to risk of overdose.

Minoxidil

Common brands
● Regaine Regular Strength (for men and women) ● Regaine Extra Strength (men only).

May prevent hereditary hair loss or promote hair growth but must be used continuously to maintain effect. Works best on small areas in younger adults with recent hair loss. New growth may take a few months.

Method of use Usually applied twice daily to clean, dry hair and scalp. Massage into scalp. Wash hands after use. Don't exceed stated dose.

Side effects Brief scalp irritation; if it persists, stop using. Hair loss may increase slightly at first.

Precautions Avoid eyes and sensitive or broken skin. *See also* GENERAL CAUTIONS, p.176.

Moisturizers

UNBRANDED: •Aqueous cream •Emulsifying ointment COMMON BRANDS: • E45 Cream (light liquid paraffin, white soft paraffin, hypoallergenic hydrous wool fat) • E45 Wash Cream (zinc oxide) • Oilatum Cream (light liquid paraffin, white soft paraffin)

Wide range of moisturizers (emollients) to soothe, soften, and help the skin retain moisture. Preparations reduce dryness, itching, and scaling, and prevent cracking and infection in problems such as psoriasis and eczema. (*See also* EMOLLIENT BATH ADDITIVES, p.181.)

Method of use Apply as often as needed, particularly after washing. Use aqueous cream or emulsifying ointment instead of soap for washing.

Side effects Rarely, sensitivity to an ingredient; stop using and contact a doctor.

Precautions None.

Mouth and throat treatments

Common brands

ANTISEPTIC MOUTHWASHES: • Colgate Chlorohex 1200 mouthwash (chlorhexidine) • Corsodyl mouthwash (chlorhexidine)
PAINKILLERS: • Dequacaine (benzocaine, dequalinium) • Difflam Sore Throat Rinse and Spray (benzydamine) • Vicks Ultra Chloraseptic (benzocaine)
BREATH FRESHENERS: • Coolmint Listerine PocketPaks • RetarDex Oral Spray

Various treatments for mouth and throat problems, such as bad breath, a sore throat, or mouth ulcers. Those containing an antiseptic help sore areas to heal and prevent further infections. Painkillers such as benzydamine help reduce pain and inflammation; local anaesthetics, such as benzocaine, numb sore areas. Fresheners give breath a pleasant smell temporarily.

Method of use Liquids used as a rinse or gargle; sprays and gels applied directly to sore areas. Throat lozenges and breath fresheners sucked or dissolved on the tongue.

Side effects Occasionally, irritation and soreness. Chlorhexidine may cause a temporary brown staining on teeth: don't use for long periods.

Precautions Gargles or throat sprays may not be suitable for children. *See also* GENERAL CAUTIONS, p.176.

Mouth ulcer treatments

Common brand
• Adcortyl in Orabase for Mouth Ulcers (triamcinolone)

Contains a steroid to reduce inflammation in a sticky base that adheres to the ulcer. (*See also* MOUTH AND THROAT TREATMENTS, below.)

Method of use Apply thinly as directed. Don't rub the paste in.

Side effects Usually none.

Precautions Don't use steroid pastes for longer than 5 days or if you have a mouth infection.

Oatmeal products

Common brand
• Aveeno cream/moisturizing lotion/bath oil

Help to soothe itchy skin caused by irritating and inflamed skin conditions.

Method of use Available as bath oils or as creams or lotions applied directly to the skin. Lotions can be used instead of soap when washing. Add bath oils to a lukewarm bath; pat skin dry.

Side effects Usually none.

Precautions Oatmeal bath additives can make the bath slippery; take care when getting in and out of the water.

Oil of cloves

Cloves (*Eugenia caryophyllata*) are traditionally used to relieve various problems, including toothache. Oil of cloves helps to numb the tooth area.

Method of use Apply a few drops to cotton wool and place directly on tooth. Be careful to keep the oil off the tongue as it may burn a little.

Side effects Usually none.

Precautions None.

Oral rehydration preparations

Common brands
• Dioralyte Relief (sodium chloride, potassium chloride, sodium citrate, precooked rice powder)
• Electrolade (sodium chloride, potassium chloride, sodium bicarbonate, dextrose)

Preparations that replace water, fluid, and salts lost from the body due to vomiting, diarrhoea, or excessive sweating.

Method of use Available as soluble powders, in many flavours, mixed with water to make a drink. Take care to add correct volume of water as directed. Use freshly boiled and cooled water when preparing for babies.

Side effects Usually none.

Precautions Consult a doctor before use if you are on a low-salt diet, have persistent vomiting, bowel blockage, diabetes, or kidney or liver problems. Check whether the product is suitable before giving to a baby.

Paracetamol

Common brands
FOR ADULTS ● Disprol ● Hedex ● Panadol
FOR CHILDREN ● Calpol Infant Suspension (3 months–6 years) ● Calpol Six Plus Fast Melts (6–12 years) ● Calpol Six Plus Suspension (6–12 years) ● Medinol Over 6 (6–12 years) ● Medinol Under 6 (3 months–6 years)

Widely used painkiller for toothache, headache, earache, muscle pains, and to reduce fever. Suitable for people with stomach problems as is less irritating than aspirin; also during breastfeeding because traces in breast milk are too small to harm a baby.

Method of use Available as regular, soluble, or melt-in-the-mouth tablets; or liquid. When treating a child, choose the correct product for child's age (*see* COMMON BRANDS, above). Infants from 2 months can be treated with Medinol under 6 and Calpol Infant Suspension for fever after vaccination, but otherwise only on doctor's advice.

Side effects Usually none.

Precautions Don't give to babies under 3 months except on a doctor's advice or to treat a fever following immunization.

WARNING
Don't take with other drugs containing painkillers and/or codeine, such as cold remedies, due to risk of overdose. In case of possible overdose, seek immediate medical attention, even if you feel no ill effects. There is risk of delayed, serious liver damage.

Paracetamol and codeine

Common brands
● Panadol Ultra ● Paracodol ● Solpadeine Max

Combination of codeine and paracetamol (*see* above) provides stronger painkilling effect than paracetamol alone. Paracetamol helps to bring down a fever.

Method of use Taken as regular or soluble tablets or as capsules.

Side effects Codeine may cause constipation; drink plenty of fluids and eat extra fibre.

Precautions May cause drowsiness or dizziness, in which case don't drive or operate machinery. *See also* GENERAL CAUTIONS, p.176.

WARNING
Don't take with other medications containing paracetamol because of risk of overdose.

Phyto-oestrogens

Natural plant chemicals, usually found in soya-based foods, that have a similar (but weaker) effect on the body to the female hormone oestrogen. Also found in flax seeds (linseed). May help to reduce menopausal symptoms such as hot flushes.

Method of use Boost diet with soya-based products, such as tofu, soya milk, and linseed bread.

Side effects Usually none if products are taken as part of a normal diet.

Precautions None.

Proton pump inhibitors

Common brand
● Zanprol (omeprazole)

Reduces amount of acid in the stomach to relieve bouts of heartburn. Initally, can be used with antacids.

Method of use Taken as a tablet that should be swallowed whole with plenty of fluids before meals. Recommended only for short-term use (no more than 4 weeks).

Side effects Usually none; may sometimes cause headaches, diarrhoea, nausea, and a rash.

Precautions Not recommended for those under 18 years. *See also* GENERAL CAUTIONS, p.176.

Salicylic acid

Common brands
● Carnation Corn Caps ● Compound W ● Scholl Polymer Gel Corn Remover ● Scholl Verruca Removal System

Salicylic acid softens hardened skin, such as calluses and corns, and warts, making them easier to remove. Available as liquids, gels, or ointments.

Method of use Make sure area is clean and dry. Wart treatment can take up to 12 weeks.

Side effects May cause mild soreness when first applied. If severe, stop using.

Precautions Avoid surrounding skin, broken or inflamed skin, moles, birth marks, warts with hair. Don't use on the face or genitals. Consult a doctor before use if you have diabetes.

Saline nose drops

These moisten the lining of nasal passages and loosen thickened mucus.

Method of use Blow your nose first. Apply a few drops into each nostril. Hold your head back for a few minutes so that the drops run inside your nose.

Side effects Usually none.

Precautions None.

Saw palmetto

A traditional remedy for men's urinary problems made from berries of saw palmetto (*Serenoa repens*). May improve urine flow and bladder emptying in men with benign (noncancerous) prostate gland enlargement.

Method of use Extracts available as tablets or capsules. Take as directed. May be several months before you notice an improvement.

Side effects Can cause stomach upsets, mild headaches, and dizziness.

Precautions Can alter results of prostate cancer screening blood tests. Discuss with a doctor first if you have any urinary problems.

Scabies and head lice lotions

Common brands
- Derbac-M (malathion) • Full Marks (phenothrin)
- Hedrin (dimeticone) • Lyclear Cream Rinse (permethrin) • Lyclear Dermal Cream (permethrin)
- Prioderm (malathion) • Quellada M (malathion)

Antiparasitic treatments for skin infestations. Malathion or permethrin (which are insecticides) for head lice and scabies mites; phenothrin (an insecticide) and dimeticone (a non-insecticide substance) only for head lice.

Method of use Insecticidal products available as shampoos or lotions in water or alcohol base. Lotions are more effective than shampoos; water-based preparations are less irritating, and preferable for scabies. Dimeticone is available as a lotion in a silicone base.

Side effects Can irritate skin. Permethrin products may also cause redness and stinging.

Precautions Avoid using insecticidal products on broken or infected skin. Avoid eyes with all products. Check suitability before using on small children or babies. Don't use alcohol-based lotions on people with asthma or eczema, or small children.

Sodium bicarbonate

Also called baking soda, commonly used in cooking. Can soothe itching and soreness.

Method of use Add 4 tablespoons (or a teacup) to a bath two-thirds full of lukewarm water and soak for about 20 minutes. For soreness inside the mouth, add half a teaspoon of sodium bicarbonate to 250 ml (half a pint) of warm water to make a mouthwash.

Side effects Usually none.

Precautions None.

Sodium cromoglicate

Common brands
- Opticrom Eye Drops • Rynacrom Nasal Spray

Nasal spray used to help prevent or relieve symptoms of hay fever and other allergic causes of runny nose. Eye drops used to relieve red, itchy eyes due to hay fever and other causes of allergic conjunctivitis, such as allergy to house dust mites.

Method of use For best results, start using nasal spray before the hay fever season begins and continue treatment through the season. Eye drops also need to be used continuously.

Side effects May briefly irritate your eyes or the lining of your nose.

Precautions Don't wear contact lenses while using the eye drops.

Steroid nasal sprays

Common brands
- Beconase Allergy (beclometasone) • Flixonase Allergy (fluticasone) • Nasobec Hayfever (beclometasone)

Contain a steroid drug that prevents or relieves hay fever attacks, and a runny nose due to other allergies, by reducing irritation and swelling in the nose. Take a few days to reach their full effect.

Method of use For best results, start using 2–3 days before exposure to allergic triggers. Use the spray every day for continual relief.

Side effects May dry and irritate nasal lining.

Precautions Don't use if you have a nasal infection. *See also* GENERAL CAUTIONS, p.176.

St John's wort

Preparations made from St John's wort (*Hypericum perforatum*), used as a remedy for mild depression.

Method of use Usually available as tablets or capsules. It is advisable to consult a doctor first before treating yourself.

Side effects Headaches, nausea, anxiety, constipation, and skin sensitivity to sunlight.

Precautions St John's wort interacts with a wide range of medications. Consult a doctor or pharmacist before use if you are taking prescribed medication. Don't use with the contraceptive pill. *See also* GENERAL CAUTIONS, p.176.

Sunscreens and sunblocks

Products designed to protect skin from harmful ultraviolet (UV) rays in sunlight. Total sunblocks (containing zinc oxide or titanium dioxide) prevent all UV light from reaching your skin. Sunscreens are graded by sun protection factor (SPF); the higher the SPF, the greater the protection.

Method of use A sunscreen with an SPF of at least 15 that protects against both UVA and UVB rays is recommended.

Side effects Sometimes, skin irritation.

Precautions Check that the product is suitable before using on a baby or child.

Threadworm treatments

Common brands
● Boots Threadworm Treatment (mebendazole)
● Ovex (mebendazole) ● Pripsen Piperazine Phosphate Powder (piperazine)

Treatments such as mebendazole or piperazine that kill worms inside the body.

Method of use Treat everyone in the household to prevent spread and/or reinfection. For adults and children over 2, give mebendazole. If reinfection occurs, a second dose after 2 weeks may be needed. For children over 3 months, give piperazine. Repeat the dose after 2 weeks.

Side effects May be abdominal pain, nausea, diarrhoea, and allergic reactions.

Precautions Consult a doctor first if a baby under 3 months has threadworms, or if you are pregnant or breastfeeding. *See also* GENERAL CAUTIONS, p.176.

WARNING
Avoid piperazine if you have epilepsy.

Travel sickness pills

Common brands
● Avomine (promethazine teoclate)
● Joy-Rides (hyoscine) ● Sea-Legs (meclozine)

Help to prevent motion sickness if taken before travelling.

Method of use Allow enough time for pills to take effect before you travel.

Side effects Some types may cause drowsiness, a dry mouth, or blurred vision.

Precautions Don't take with alcohol. If drowsy, don't drive or use hazardous machinery.

Vitamin B$_6$ (pyridoxine)

Supplements of vitamin B$_6$, or boosting the diet with foods rich in the vitamin, may help prevent PMS, and also cyclical breast pain and/or lumpiness.

Method of use Available as capsules. May need to be taken for 2–3 months to benefit. Foods containing B$_6$ include poultry, fish, eggs, soya, oats, wholegrain products, bananas, and nuts.

Side effects Usually none.

Precautions Don't exceed the recommended dose; high doses may cause nerve damage.

Wart and verruca treatments

Common brands
SALICYLIC ACID: ● Boots Verruca Removal Gel
● Scholl Verruca Removal System
FREEZERS: ● Scholl Freeze Wart & Verruca Remover
● Wartner Verruca Remover ● Wartner Wart Remover

Salicylic acid softens warts and verrucas so that they are easier to remove. Freezers freeze warts and verrucas to the core, making them fall off.

Method of use For salicylic acid, make sure the area is clean and dry and apply a small amount to the wart. Repeat applications are usually needed before the wart disappears. For freezers, spray on the medication or use the applicator. A single treatment may be effective within 10–14 days, although repeat treatments may be needed.

Side effects Both types of treatment may cause redness, soreness, or stinging when applied.

Precautions For both treatments, avoid normal skin, broken or inflamed skin, moles, birth marks, and warts with hair. Freezers should not be used under the age of 4. Consult a doctor before use if you have diabetes or are pregnant or breastfeeding.

Index

A

Abdominal problems 106–18
  bloating and flatulence 108
  constipation 115
  diarrhoea 116, 136, 143
  food intolerance 113
  food poisoning 114
  heartburn 107
  hernia 112
  indigestion 106
  irritable bowel syndrome 111
  itchy anus 118
  motion sickness 110
  nausea and vomiting 109, 136, 143
  piles 117
Achilles tendon 99
Aciclovir 177
Acne 37
Air travel 18, 66, 96
Airway, choking 172–3
Allergies
  anaphylactic shock 159
  blocked or runny nose 77
  conjunctivitis 58
  eczema 38
  hay fever 80
  hives 36
  itchy eyes 56
  wheezing 103
Aloe vera 177
Aluminium chloride 177
Anaphylactic shock 159
Ankles, swollen 96
Antacids 177
Anti-dandruff shampoos 177
Antidiarrhoeal drugs 177
Antifungal drugs 178
Antihistamines 178
Anti-nailbiting lotions 178
Antispasmodic drugs 178
Anus
  itchy anus 118
  piles 117
  threadworms 137
Arms
  fractures 161
  tennis or golfer's elbow 91
Aromatic oils 178
Arthritis 92, 93
Aspirin 179
Athlete's foot 44

B

Babies 142–53
  choking 173
  colic 148
  CPR 171
  cradle cap 151

  crying 149
  diarrhoea and vomiting 143
  feeding problems 144–5
  fever 142
  heat rash 46
  nappy rash 152
  recovery position 169
  rescue breathing 171
  settling 149
  sleep problems 146–7
  spots, rashes, and skin problems 150
Back pain 88–9
Bad breath 72
Baths
  emollient additives 181
  salt-water 120
Bed, safety getting out of 88
Bedwetting 139
Benzoyl peroxide 179
Bites, insect 158
Black eye 62
Blackheads 37
Bladder
  cystitis 130
  men's urinary problems 121
  poor control 131
Bleeding
  cuts and grazes 156
  gums 74
  nosebleed 83
  severe 157
Blepharitis 56
Blisters 155
Bloating 108
Boils 45
Bones, fractures 161
Bottle-feeding 144, 145
Bowels
  constipation 115
  diarrhoea 116, 136, 143
  irritable bowel syndrome 111
Breastfeeding 125, 126, 144–5
Breasts
  breast awareness 125
  breast pain and lumpy breasts 124–5
  cracked nipples 126
Breathing
  rebreathing into a paper bag 24, 101
  reducing stress 20
  rescue breathing 170–1
  wheezing 103
Broken bones 161
Bronchitis 104
Bunions 98
Burns 164
Bursitis 92, 93

C

Calamine lotion 179
Calendula cream 179
Calluses 42
Cardiopulmonary resuscitation (CPR) 170–1
Chapped lips 69
Chemicals, in eye 163
Chest compressions 170–1
Chest problems 101–5
  bronchitis 104
  coughing 102
  hiccups 101
  palpitations 105
  wheezing 103
Chickenpox 32
Children's problems 135–41
  bedwetting 139
  choking 173
  CPR 171
  croup 138
  diarrhoea and vomiting 136
  earache 140
  febrile seizures 167
  fever 135
  recovery position 169
  rescue breathing 171
  temper tantrums 141
  threadworms 137
Chloramphenicol 179
Choking 172–3
Chondroitin 182
Cloves, oil of 186
Coal tar preparations 179
Codeine 187
Cold fingers and toes 100
Colds 77, 78
  remedies 179
Cold sores 70
Colic 148
Combing, head lice 50
Compresses, warm 45, 59, 64
Conjunctivitis 58
Consciousness, loss of 168–9
Constipation 115
Contact lens problems 60
Convulsions 166
Corns 42
Coughing 102
  acute bronchitis 104
  cough suppressants 180
  croup 138
Counter-irritants 180
CPR (cardiopulmonary resuscitation) 170–1
Cradle cap 151
Cramps, leg 94
Crotamiton preparations 180
Croup 138

Crying, babies 147, 148, 149
Cuts 156
Cystitis 130, 180

D

Dandruff 49
Deafness 63, 64, 66, 67, 68
Decongestants 181
Deep vein thrombosis 96
Depression 22–3
Diarrhoea 116
  babies 143
  children 136
Diet
  boosting immune system 28, 37
  elimination 113
Digestive problems
  bloating and flatulence 108
  constipation 115
  diarrhoea 116, 136, 143
  food intolerance 113
  food poisoning 114
  heartburn 107
  indigestion 106
  irritable bowel syndrome 111
  motion sickness 110
  nausea and vomiting 109, 136, 143
Diseases, infectious 26–33
Dislocation, joints 161
Dizziness 19
Dry skin 41

E

Ears
  earache 64, 140
  foreign objects in 68
  popping ears 66
  swimmer's ear 65
  tinnitus 67
  wax in 63, 181
Echinacea 181
Eczema 38
Ejaculation, premature 123
Elbow, tennis or golfer's 91
Elimination diet 113
Emergency action plan 154
Emollient bath additives 181
Epilepsy 166
Erectile dysfunction (impotence) 122
Essential fatty acids (EFAs) 181
Exercises
  calf stretches 94
  elbow stretches 91
  feet 98
  in-flight 96
  neck 87
  pelvic floor 131
  shoulder 90

Eyes
black eye 62
conjunctivitis 58
contact lens problems 60
dry eyes 57
foreign bodies in 61
injuries 163
itchy eyes 56
lubricants 181
styes 59

F
Fainting 19
Febrile seizures 167
Feeding problems, babies 144–5
Feet
athlete's foot 44
blisters 155
bunions 98
cold toes 100
corns and calluses 42
exercises 96, 98
heel pain 99
ingrowing toenails 55
pain in 97
verrucas 43
Fever 12
babies 142
children 135
Feverfew 182
Fingers, cold 100
First aid 154–74
Fits 166
Flatulence 108, 182
Flu 30
remedies 179
Food intolerance 113
Food poisoning 114
Foreign objects
choking 172–3
in the ear 68
in the eye 61
splinters 156
Fractures 161
Fungal infections
athlete's foot and jock itch 44
nails 53

G
Gastroenteritis 109, 136, 143
Genital irritation 133
German measles (rubella) 27
Ginger 182
Gingivitis 74
Glandular fever 28, 81
Glucosamine 182
Grazes 156
Gums, bleeding 74

H
H2-blockers 182
Haemorrhoids 117, 182
Hair
bleaches 183
dandruff 49

hair removal products 183
head lice 50
thinning and loss of 52
unwanted or ingrowing 51
Halitosis 72
Hangover 16, 183
Hay fever 56, 80
Headache 85
Head injuries 162
Head lice 50, 188
Hearing loss 63, 64, 66, 67, 68
Heart
CPR 170–1
palpitations 105
Heartburn 107
Heat rash 46–7
Heel pain 99
Herbal sleeping remedies 183
Herbal teas 183
Hernia 112
Herpes simplex virus 70
Hiccups 101
Hip pain 92
Hives 36
Hoarseness 82
Humidifiers 31
Hydrocolloid plasters 183
Hydrocortisone cream 184
Hygiene 136, 143
food 114
oral 74
threadworms 137

I
Ibuprofen 184
Ice packs 62
Immunization 27, 29, 30, 31
Impetigo 34
Impotence (erectile dysfunction) 122
Incontinence 131
Indigestion 106
Infectious diseases 26–33
Influenza 30
remedies 179
Inhalation, steam 79, 138
Insects
bites and stings 158, 184
in ears 68
Insomnia see Sleep problems
Irritable bowel syndrome 111
Itching 14
anus 118
eyes 56
genital irritation 133
scabies 35

J, K, L
Jet lag 18
Jock itch 44
Joints
dislocations 161
sprains 160
Knee pain 93
Lactase supplements 184
Lanolin ointment 184

Laryngitis 82
Lavender 184
Laxatives 185
Legs
cramps 94
fractures 161
swollen ankles 96
varicose veins 95
Lice, head 50, 188
Ligaments, sprains 160
Lips
chapped or cracked 69
creams, balms, and salves 185
Lubricating jelly 185
Lungs
acute bronchitis 104
coughing 102
wheezy chest 103

M
Mastitis 125
Measles 29
Memory problems 25
Meningitis 150
Menopausal problems 129
Men's problems 119–23
erectile dysfuncton (impotence) 122
painful penis 120
painful scrotum 119
premature ejaculation 123
urinary problems 121
Menstruation see Periods
Migraine 86
remedies 185
Minoxidil 185
Moisturizers 186
Motion sickness 110, 189
Mouth problems 69–76
bad breath 72
bleeding gums 74
chapped or cracked lips 69
cold sores 70
knocked-out tooth 76
sensitive teeth 75
sore mouth or tongue 73
swallowed poisons 174
toothache 75
treatments 186
ulcers 73, 186
Mumps 26
Muscles
leg cramps 94
relaxation 21
strains 160

N
Nails
biting 54, 178
disfigured or brittle 53
ingrowing toenails 55
Napping, power 15
Nappy rash 152
Nasal sprays, steroid 188
Nasal strips, snoring remedy 84

Nausea 109
motion sickness 110
Neck, sore or stiff 87
Nipples
breastfeeding 144
cracked nipples 126
Nits 50
Nose problems 77–80
blocked or runny nose 77
common cold 78
hay fever 80
nosebleed 83
saline nose drops 187
sinusitis 79
snoring 84

O, P
Oatmeal products 186
Oestrogen 187
Oil of cloves 186
Oils, aromatic 178
Oral hygiene 74
Oral rehydration products 186
Otitis externa 65
Pain
back 88–9
breast 124–5
foot 97
headaches 85
heel 99
hips 92
intercourse 134
knee 93
leg cramps 94
migraine 86
periods 128
scrotum 119
shoulder 90
tennis or golfer's elbow 91
Painkillers 179, 184, 187
Palpitations 105
Panic attacks 24
Paracetamol 187
Paracetamol and codeine 187
Pelvic floor exercises 131
Pelvis, fractures 161
Penis
erectile dysfunction (impotence) 122
painful penis 120
premature ejaculation 123
squeeze technique 123
Periods
painful 128
premenstrual syndrome 127
Phyto-oestrogens 187
Piles 117
Poisons, swallowed 174
Popping ears 66
Premature ejaculation 123
Premenstrual syndrome (PMS) 127
Prickly heat 46–7
Prostate gland 121
Proton pump inhibitors 187
Psoriasis 39

R

Rashes
babies 150
chickenpox 32
heat rash 46–7
hives 36
measles 29
meningitis 150
nappy rash 152
rosacea 40
rubella 27
shingles 33
Raynaud's disease 100
Recovery position 169
Reflux 144, 145
Rehydration, oral 186
Relaxation 21
Rescue breathing 170
R.I.C.E. procedure 160
Ringworm 48
Rosacea 40
Rubella 27

S

Safety
lifting 112
in the sun 47
Salicylic acid 187
Saline nose drops 188
Saw palmetto 188
Scabies 35, 188
Scrotum, painful 119
Seasonal affective disorder
(SAD) 23
Seizures 166
Sex
erectile dysfunction (impotence)
122
painful intercourse 134
premature ejaculation 123
Shampoo, anti-dandruff 177

Shingles 33
Shock 165
anaphylactic 159
Shoulder pain 90
Sinusitis 79
Skin problems 34–48
babies 150, 152
blisters 155
burns and scalds 164
cuts, grazes, and splinters 156
itching 14
Sleep problems 17
babies 146–7
heartburn 107
herbal remedies 183
Slings 161
Snoring 84
Sodium bicarbonate 188
Sodium cromoglicate 188
Sore mouth 73
Sore throat 81
Splinters 156
Sprains 160
Squeeze technique 123
Steroid nasal sprays 188
Stings, insect 158
St John's wort 189
Strains 160
Stress 20–1
Stress incontinence 131
Stye 59
Sunburn 46–7
Sunscreens and sunblocks 189
Sweating, excessive 13
Swimmer's ear 65
Swollen ankles 96

T

Teeth
knocked-out tooth 76
oral hygiene 74

sensitive teeth 75
toothache 75
Temperature, fever 12, 135, 142
Temper tantrums 141
Tendons
strains 160
tendinitis 91, 99
Tennis elbow 91
Testicles, self-examination 119
Thermometers 12, 135
Threadworms 137, 189
Throat problems
coughing 102
hoarseness and loss of
voice 82
sore throat 81
swallowed poisons 174
Thrombosis, deep vein 96
Tinnitus 67
Tiredness 15
Toenails
cutting 55
ingrowing 55
Toes
bunions 98
cold toes 100
Tongue, sore 73
Tonsillitis 81
Toothache 75
Travel sickness 110, 189

U, V

Ulcer, mouth 71
Unconsciousness 168–9
Urinary problems
bedwetting 139
cystitis 130
men's problems 121
women's problems: poor bladder
control 131
Urticaria (hives) 36

Vagina
discharge 132
genital irritation 133
Varicose veins 95
Veins
piles 117
varicose veins 95
Verrucas 43
Vitamin B$_6$ 189
Voice, loss of 82
Vomiting 109
babies 143
children 136
food poisoning 114
motion sickness 110, 189

W

Wart and verruca treatments 189
Warts 43
Wax, in ears 63, 181
Waxing, hair removal 51
Wheezing 103
Whooping cough 31
Women's problems 124–34
bladder control 131
breast pain and lumpy breasts
124–5
cracked nipples 126
cystitis 130
genital irritation 133
menopausal problems 129
painful intercourse 134
painful periods 128
premenstrual syndrome 127
vaginal discharge 132
Wounds, first aid 156

Y, Z

Yoghurt 132
Zinc and castor oil cream 152
Zinc lozenges 78

Acknowledgments

I am indebted to my wife Ann for her unstinting support and encouragement and especially for her expert writing and contributions to the articles in the baby and child sections.

I would also like to thank friends and colleagues for their help and encouragement, especially Martin Dunitz, Josephine Lawson of the Josephine Lawson Physiotherapy Clinic, London, and Harry Ganz of The Garden Pharmacy, London. I would also like to thank Mr David Abrams, Drs Ian and Tanya Beider, Mr Amir Kaisary, Irving Lancer, Dr Fred Lim, Dr Colin McDougall, Mr Alan Naftalin, Menachem Salasnik, Dr Lester Sireling, Dr Richard Teller, and Dr Bernard Valman.

Dorling Kindersley would like to thank:
Project photography: Gary Ombler
Additional photography: Peter Andersona, Jake Fitzjones, and Esther Ripley
Jacket designers: Mark Cavanagh, Matthew Robbins
Index: Hilary Bird
Proofreader: Alyson Lacewing
First aid validated by Jemima Dunne
Models: Ann Baggaley, Babita Bholah, Angela Cameron, Steve Capon, Gary Harding, Karen Heaton, Rosalie Hunt, Jo Lyford, Shahid Mahmood, Freya Mahony, Charlotte Mahony, Tony Maine, Brian North, Benji Peters, Morgan Steel, Duncan Steel, Shelia Tait, Scott Totman, Jeremy Wallis.
Picture Credits: (abbreviations key: t=top, r=right)
The Ivy Press Ltd/Guy Ryecart **p.17**; Allergy-matters Ltd (www.allergymatters.com) **p.23**; Science Photo Library/ John Radcliffe Hospital (tr) **p.29**; Science Photo Library/Eamonn McNulty

(tr) **p.32**; Science Photo Library/Biophoto Associates **p.33**; St John's Institute of Dermatology **p.34**; Science Photo Library/Dr P. Marazzi (tr) **p.35**; Dr D. A. Burns **p.38**; Dr D. A. Burns (tr) **p.39**; Science Photo Library/CNRI **p.40**; Science Photo Library/Dr P. Marazzi **p.42**; Science Photo Library (tr) **p.44**; Science Photo Library **p.48**; Science Photo Library/Dr Chris Hale (tr) **p.50**; Science Photo Library/Sue Ford (tr) **p.59**; Science Photo Library/St Bartholomew's Hospital (tr) **p.70**; Science Photo Library/Dr P. Marazzi **p.71**; Getty Images/Vicky Kasala Productions **p.92**; Science Photo Library **p.95**; Science Photo Library/ Dr P. Marazzi (tr) **p.98**; Nauticalia Ltd **p.100**; Photofusion/Clarissa Leahy **p.145**; Mother & Baby Picture Library/ EMAP **p.146**; Getty/Photodisc **p.147**; Meningitis Research Foundation **p.150**; Science Photo Library/Chris Priest (tr) **p.151**.

All other images © Dorling Kindersley.
For further information see: www.dkimages.com